The CORE Kettlebell Challenge

40 Days to Lose Fat, Improve Performance, Change Your Mind and Change Your Life

Published By Forest Vance Training Inc.
1530 X Street, Sacramento, CA 95818
ForestVance.com

Editor: Stacey Lenn (a.k.a. Grammargal)

Photography: Aniko Kinzel

Cover Design: Hisna Nur Azizah

Interior Design: Chinthaka Wijebahu aka cebooker

Library of Congress Cataloging-in-Publication Data
Vance, Forest
ISBN 9781710559422
1. Strength Training
2. Fitness
3. Physical education and training.

ADVANCE PRAISE FOR THE CORE KETTLEBELL CHALLENGE

"One of the most important things you need to truly transform your body is a 'reason why.' Forest tells you his . . . and he will help you find YOURS. And then he'll give you the exact plan and tools you need to make it happen. This book lays it all out for you in an easy-to-understand, actionable manner. Highly recommended."

—**Nick Nilsson**, **http://www.madscientistofmuscle.com**

"Forest has a unique and compelling perspective to get you fit mentally and physically. He took his experience of connecting with amazing strength and conditioning coaches during his NFL tenure, his personal journey of losing over sixty pounds, and his incredible resume including dozens of certifications, and put it all in this book. It's no wonder his transformation clients rave about him. They physically and mentally upgraded their lives, and you will too."

—**Mike Whitfield**, Author and Master CTT

"The fitness industry is largely broken. Thankfully we have some people like Forest Vance that can take an overly-complicated subject and distill it down to what works. Forest has done it himself, and he has coached hundreds of students for lasting results in building strength, moving better, losing fat, and feeling better. The CORE Kettlebell Challenge is an effective program to help you do the same."

—**Logan Christopher**, Founder of Legendary Strength and Lost Empire Herbs

Disclaimer

Strenuous physical exercise can be a dangerous activity. There are inherent risks in any physical activity, and intense fitness training is no exception. The use of professional instruction is recommended before entering into any type of sport or physical exercise. You should become knowledgeable about the risks involved and assume personal responsibility for your actions. The information contained within this manual may or may not be accurate and is open to interpretation.

For my wife, Gina.
This book wouldn't exist without your love and support.

TABLE OF CONTENTS

INTRODUCTION

Are you looking for a new challenge to change your routine, shake things up, and kick it up a notch?

Do you want to bust your current plateau, get more done in less time, and take your training to the next level?

Are you just looking for a new reason to get excited about your workouts again?

I believe that if you answered yes to the questions above, I have the perfect solution to help you lose fat, gain muscle, increase energy, and get it back—in just forty days.

It's called the CORE (Challenge-Oriented, Results-Earned) Kettlebell Challenge.

My name is Forest Vance.

In a former life, I was a pro football player.

Over the last fourteen years, I've worked in many different roles as a trainer and coach in the world of health and fitness.

This book is the sum total of my life's work, which includes the following:

- Twenty-four years of my own personal training experience, including exposure to some of the top strength and conditioning coaches in the world during my time in the NFL
- Fourteen years of in-the-trenches training experience, and over 16,000 client sessions
- A Master's Degree in Human Movement
- Eighteen general and specialty training certifications
- Hundreds of books read, DVDs watched, and home study courses taken

I can promise you results if you follow my lead.

It's not going to be easy, but it will be worth it.

Together, over the next forty days, we're going to help you become the strongest version of yourself.

Forest Vance
August 12, 2019
Sacramento, CA

PART 1:

KETTLEBELLS! - THE ULTIMATE TOOL FOR FAT LOSS AND PERFORMANCE

It is not the critic who counts; not the man who points out how the strong man stumbles, or where the doer of deeds could have done them better. The credit belongs to the man who is actually in the arena, whose face is marred by dust and sweat and blood; who strives valiantly; who errs, who comes short again and again, because there is no effort without error and shortcoming; but who does actually strive to do the deeds; who knows great enthusiasms, the great devotions; who spends himself in a worthy cause; who at the best knows in the end the triumph of high achievement, and who at the worst, if he fails, at least fails while daring greatly, so that his place shall never be with those cold and timid souls who neither know victory nor defeat.

—Theodore Roosevelt; Paris, France; April 23, 1910

ATHLETE VS. INNER FAT KID

Almost every personal trainer I've met falls into one of two categories:

1. They have an athletic background and a love for physical training and want to help others see the same benefits they have.
2. They underwent a physical and mental transformation themselves and now want to help others do the same.

I actually fall into both.

I played sports from a young age and have always been a good athlete. I was a three-time All-American football player at the University of California at Davis and played for a couple of years in the NFL.

But also, since I can remember, my weight has been up and down.

As an adult, I've managed to keep it pretty stable for the last thirteen or fourteen years . . . but it's taken a lot of work to get here.

In this first section of the CORE Kettlebell Challenge, I'm going to share with you stories of my love of strength from a young age, my evolution as an athlete, struggles I've had along the way, and the solution that's helped me get fit, strong, and healthy - and <u>stay</u> there.

MY FIRST SET OF WEIGHTS

I remember being six or seven years old and wanting a set of weights really badly.

My mom wouldn't let me have them because she thought it might be bad for me to lift at such a young age.

But a family friend gave some to me as a gift, so my mom relented and let me have them.

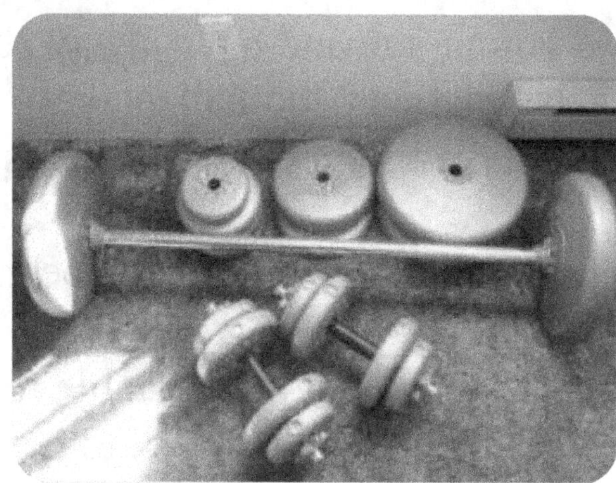

I remember doing exercises from the booklet that was included with the weight set, and I thought it was about the coolest thing ever. What seven-year-old kid gets excited about lifting weights?

Looking back, it's obvious to me that physical training and learning how to develop my body and mind was a passion from a very young age.

ADDICTED TO THE PUMP

Flash forward to the age of thirteen.

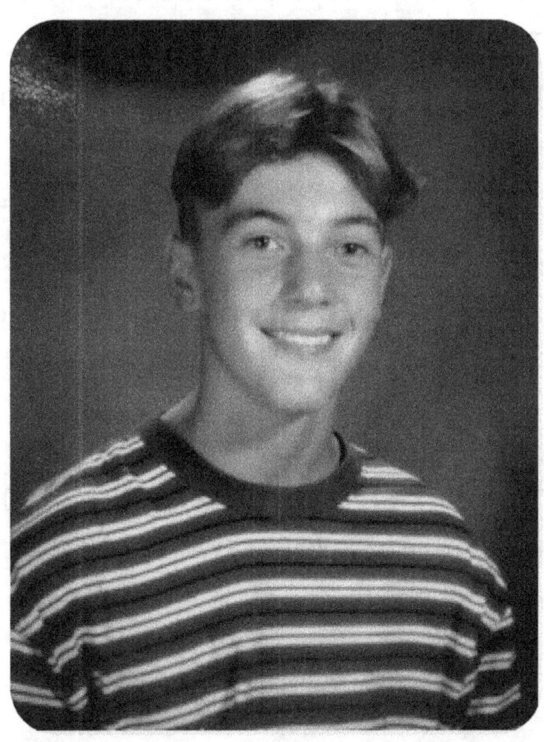

I was a decent athlete. I played baseball and basketball all through grade school and was typically one of the better players on teams I was on.

I also remember liking the conditioning and calisthenics we did, but I was always in the minority. The other kids hated it. But I saw it as an opportunity to get better, even then.

One morning when I was visiting my grandma in Southern California and getting ready to head out to the beach, I decided I would do some push-ups and sit-ups.

I looked in the mirror when I was done with the set and could see that my chest and abs looked different, instantly.

I was looking good and feeling good and ready to set out in my swim trunks and find some lucky ladies.

From that day on, I was hooked on the feeling working out gives you— what's called the "pump." (What's happening here from a physiological standpoint is that blood rushes into the muscle group(s) you are training. You get a really tight feeling like your muscles are going to explode any minute, like an over-stretched water balloon. It feels fantastic!)

Now the pump may feel good in the short term. Research is not conclusive as to whether it actually results in long-term gains - which is why it's not a focus of the CORE Kettlebell Challenge program (Shoenfeld & Contreras, 2014). Still, this early experience was a pivotal moment, and it led to increased interest in strength training for me moving forward.

LEARNING TO LIFT

The year after I turned thirteen, the very first thing our freshman year, I remember testing out the bench press.

I did 115. Not exactly spectacular.

I was six foot three and about 160 pounds.

And I wasn't the best athlete that year either—I didn't even earn a starting spot on my freshman football team.

But the next year I filled out, gained 30 pounds and a lot of strength, and was suddenly a force to be reckoned with.

I owe a lot of that to hitting the weights and starting to learn how to train my body.

Over the next couple of years, I developed a lot and became a very good football player and track athlete.

We had a lift-a-thon my junior year where we power cleaned as much as we could to raise money for the football program. I did three hundred pounds—another product of my hard work in the weight room—and attracted attention from college scouts.

I am naturally a good athlete. But I believe my hard work in the weight room and on the field in the off-season was also a big part of my success through the years, and what led me to where I am today.

MY INNER NERD

Most of my friends at sixteen and seventeen were spending their summers down at the river and/or drinking beers and/or chasing girls.

I did a little bit of all of these activities. But I also loved physical training. I remember spending my summers lifting weights for hours at the gym, out on the track doing extra conditioning, and reading and learning all I could on the topic of improving my body.

Back in those days, the muscle magazines, some books, and a handful of websites were what we had to go on.

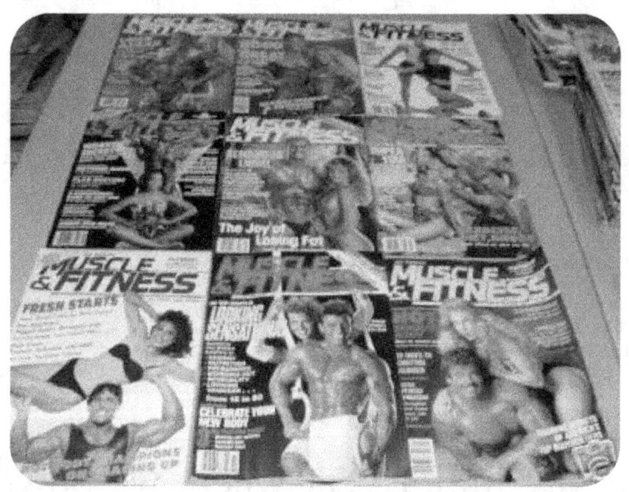

There were just a few reputable websites where you could get quality information.

Message boards were also very popular, but you never knew if you could trust the info on them.

Even though I didn't learn about kettlebell training until years later, what I learned in these early days formed the foundation of knowledge that ended up going into this book.

HIGH SCHOOL SENIOR PROJECT

I loved training so much that I did my senior project in high school on exercise.

I put together a program—a training and diet plan to gain muscle—and used myself as the test subject.

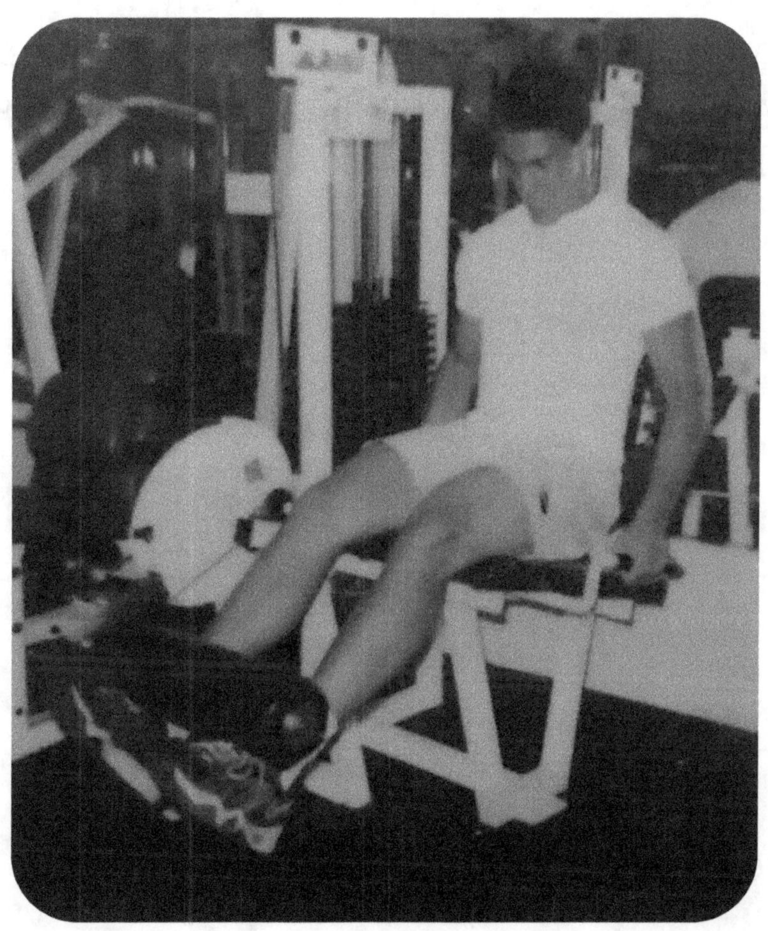

To my surprise, I ended up putting on five pounds of muscle over six weeks.

This is when I actually start thinking that eventually I might be in the fitness field as a profession, as a strength coach or something similar.

COLLEGE FOOTBALL DAYS

I ended up getting a scholarship to play football at the University of California at Davis.

I was a little bit disappointed, because I had been recruited by some bigger schools, but it didn't end up working out.

However, this turned out to be a blessing. Davis was a perfect fit. I got the opportunity to start every single game of my college career, from freshman to senior year. I never missed a game!

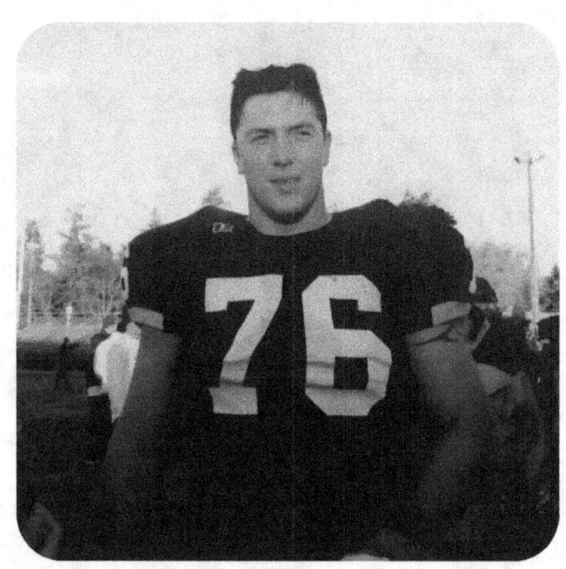

I also was a three-time All-American.

Throughout my college football career, my love of physical training persisted. Lifting weights was a huge passion, and I spent my extra time writing workout plans, doing the ones we did for football, *and* doing my own. I worked in a supplement store so I could get a discount on the products and learn more about health and fitness.

THE NFL

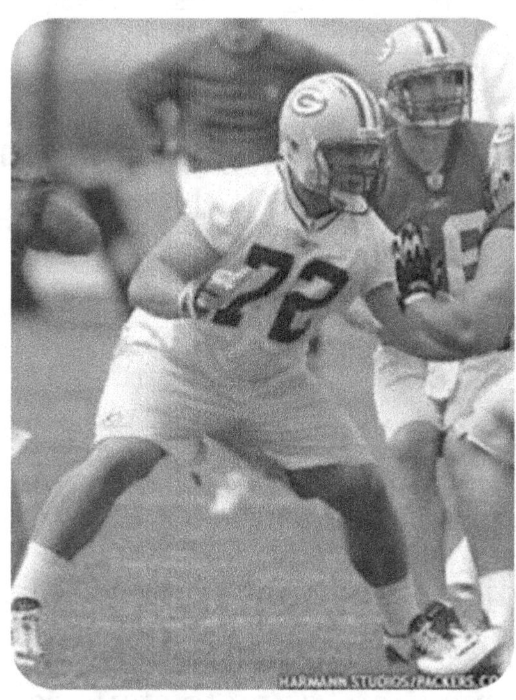

Then I got the chance to play pro football for about two years.

It was an amazing experience that I will never forget.

Right out of college, I got to go to Green Bay.

Brett Farve was standing right there in the locker room next to me on my first day as I was about to get my physical, cracking jokes and giving the rookies a hard time. I was so starstruck.

I was in Green Bay from the first mini-camp right after the draft, right up into training camp.

I injured my knee in training camp that year and ended up needing surgery and getting waived injured. I was very disappointed because I knew that could have been my one shot to make an NFL team.

That was really one of the first down times in my life. I felt like my life had been rolling along and going along exactly as I thought it would, and then I got thrown a huge curveball.

Things won't always go exactly as planned in your life journey. But the important thing to understand is that there IS a greater plan. And that God's got this.

So I headed home to the Sacramento, California, area and got back to training. I wanted to try to rehab my knee and get to feeling better and back in shape so I could get on another NFL team.

I spent the next eight months getting another knee surgery, then a hand surgery for another injury that I didn't even realize I had, and working odd jobs while at the same time trying to stay prepared and ready in case I got a call to come out for an NFL team.
I ended up getting a few different tryouts with different teams, and they didn't work out—I failed one physical and another tryout got canceled at the last minute.

But then I got a call from Kansas City. They liked what they saw, and they offered me a contract.

I got the chance to play again!

So I moved to KC and spent the next four months there.

It was another great experience.

This time I ended up getting released early in training camp, and again was sent packing.

Now after bouncing around from one team to another and going through all I've outlined for you here, I weighed my options carefully.

Sometimes you have to sit and look at your future and pray and figure out what to do with your life.

I decided to move on and retire from football and go on to the next phase of my life.

That takes us to the next part of this book, where my big physical transformation took place and I ended up becoming a personal trainer.

HOW I LOST 64 POUNDS IN SEVEN MONTHS

Now here I was. After a fourteen-year football career, including two years in the NFL, I had "retired" . . . and within a matter of months found myself *very* out of shape.

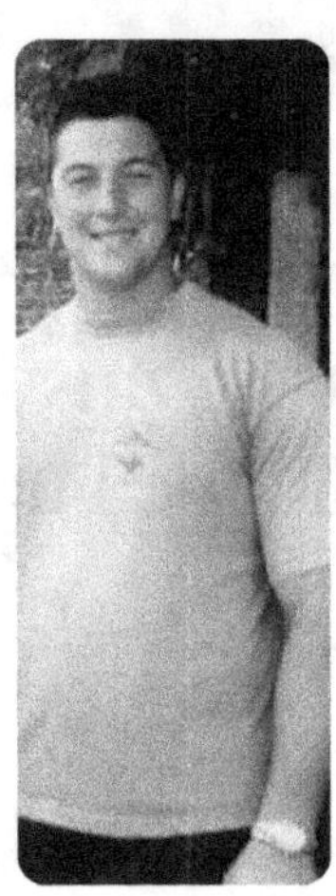

I really wanted to trim down and get healthy, but as strange as it sounds, I wasn't sure where to start.

The new goals I had were quite different from what I had trained for throughout my athletic career.

I didn't want to get ripped and jacked as much as I wanted to lean down, feel great, and be healthy.

And although I was SUPER disciplined during my athletic career . . . for various reasons, I had slipped out of good habits and fallen into some not-so-good ones.

So I learned, I researched . . . I read every book and watched every DVD I could get my hands on . . .

I put what I learned to work, and I ended up losing sixty-four pounds in seven months.

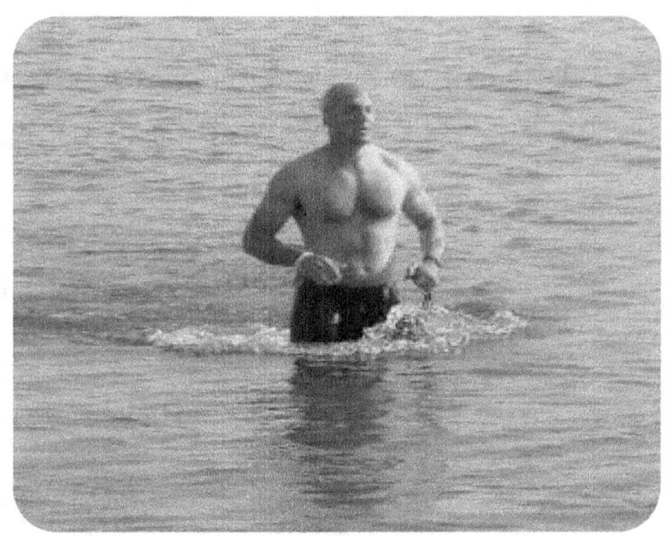

I've managed to keep the weight off over fifteen years later. And my personal fitness journey put me on the path of writing of this book . . .

A TWO-HOUR WORKOUT – IN TWENTY MINUTES

You see, one huge factor I think that got me so out of shape—and this is also true for so many clients I work with—is that as life progresses, you have <u>less time</u>.

When I was nineteen years old, I often slept late, went to class, worked a part-time job, studied, and still had hours of extra time each day. If I wanted to work out for two hours, I easily could.

We used to go to the gym. Do cardio. Then lift. Then do abs. Then stretch.

Today, that would be almost impossible. With working fifty hours per week and running businesses and a young family and church life and so much more, squeezing thirty minutes per day is about all I can do.

But fortunately, I discovered kettlebells.

They are the ultimate tool for getting a lot done in a short amount of time.

Now, in about twenty minutes, using the high intensity intervals combined with resistance training that you can get with kettlebells, I can get as good of a workout or even better than I used to in two hours (Foster, Farland, Guidotti et all, 2015).

And that's what the CORE Kettlebell Challenge program is all about.

PERFORMANCE AND RESULTS

Now, when I first started my weight loss journey, my #1 goal was weight loss. So I knew I needed to design my workouts around that goal.

But the main focus of my workouts up to that point in time had been performance.

That is, I wasn't just training for weight loss or to hit a certain number of inches gone. Every time I hit the gym, it was to put a few more pounds on the squat bar, or add a couple reps to the bench press.

This performance-based concept—setting goals like doing a few more reps of push-ups or squats in a certain amount of time, etc.—really accelerated my results and actually helped me make progress and eventually reach my weight loss goal, but in a fun and enjoyable way.

And so, this performance-based idea, as you'll see shortly, is a big part of the CORE Kettlebell Challenge.

WHAT TO EXPECT

The real magic lies in the way we combine this concept of performance-based workouts and kettlebells. That's why the program is called CORE: Challenge-Oriented, Results-Earned.

Kettlebells are the perfect tool to incorporate into this style of workout for an extra challenge. Even better, these workouts take around twenty minutes to complete, and can be done with just a single kettlebell and your own body weight.

This is the method I have created and used with my clients to help them achieve amazing success.

Here are a few of the benefits you can expect when you try out this full system for yourself:

- Slashed body fat
- Lean, athletic-looking build
- Ability to lift more weight
- Tightened up body
- Strength—without lots of expensive equipment
- Quicker workout that can fit into your crazy schedule
- Decreased strain on your body—so you can get into the best shape of your life without beating yourself up and getting all these little tweaks and injuries
- Seamless integration of kettlebells and body weight, improving the efficiency and effectiveness of your kettlebell routine

KETTLEBELL SUCCESS STORIES

I want to showcase a few of my top students from the last few years.

These men and women have achieved tremendous success with my kettlebell training methods.

As you'll see, they each came to me with unique situations and challenges.

But each of their stories is very relatable. I think you'll read them and move forward thinking, "If they can do it, I can do it too!"

I also think these stories will ease any concerns you might have before starting the program.

KEITH LOST 40+ POUNDS

We had opened the doors of our new fitness and performance facility just three days prior. Keith walked into the gym, and the second I introduced myself to him, I knew he was committed and ready to make a change . . . but he had no plan.

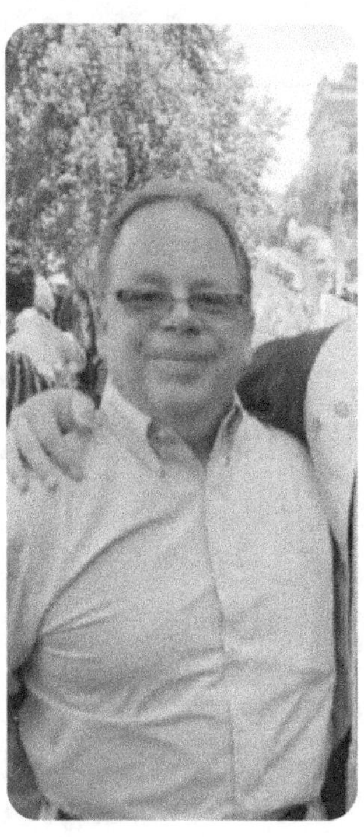

He told me in our recent interview: *"I knew that I had to lose weight and make a change for my health . . . but I didn't know where exactly to start."*

We sat down for an intro session the next day, mapped out the plan he would need to follow for the next twelve months to reach his goals, and got started right away working toward them together.

Keith has been one of our most committed and consistent clients ever since that first day. He is happily married with three children and is actively involved with the activities and responsibilities that brings. He also works in his family business, travels all around Northern California, and works long and hard hours—but he makes his fitness program a priority. He makes time and gets in and gets it done, four times per week, no matter what.

Keith says:

"The only way you'll see a difference is if you make a commitment to yourself and stick to it."

In the last twenty-two months we've worked together, Keith has met his initial weight loss goal and surpassed it. He's down a total of forty pounds—and just a few weeks ago, he completed the Spartan Beast, a 15+ mile, 35+ obstacle race, done at elevation in Lake Tahoe.

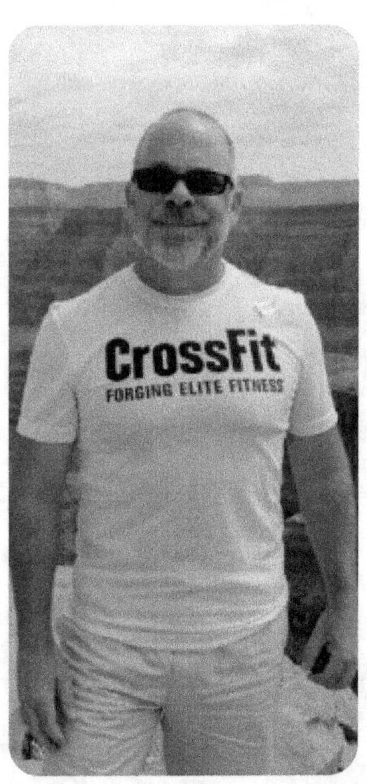

"When I started at FVT at the age of 51, I never thought I would be able to do some of the things I've accomplished here. I'd say I'm in the best shape of my life, and I'm still just as excited about training at FVT as I was the first day I walked in. It's never too late to start your fitness journey!"

Keith's amazing transformation is proof that with commitment and dedication, the results will follow!

PAM LOST 50+ POUNDS

Pam wrote her entire story and gave us permission to publish it here. Read it below; I know you will be inspired:

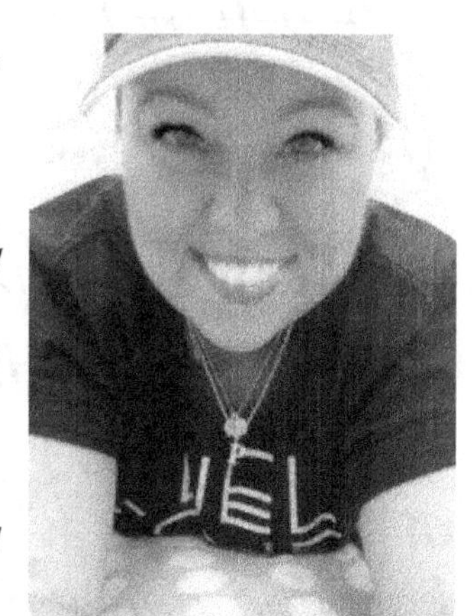

"I was working, trying to have kids, trying to have it all.

I gained a ton of weight during fertility treatments and trying to have biological children. (We adopted the best kids I could have ever hoped for!)

However, I never really addressed my weight gain and what to do about it. And as anyone with kids knows, kid diets are very different from your pre-kid diets.

And . . . I LOVE food . . . and carbs. My whole family loves food and especially sugary, carb-heavy foods. They made me feel happy (and probably still do!).

I hadn't even realized how much weight I had gained on my five foot one frame until most of my clothes in my closet weren't fitting anymore. Then I was depressed, and that came with its own host of diet and exercise problems. I didn't know where to start. Once my scale hit 180 pounds, I knew something HAD to change.

So I always tell anyone who will listen: just start walking. Then running, even if just for a minute, then increase by a minute a week. And just don't buy unhealthy snacks or sugars to keep at home—if you don't have them, you will have to get up, go out, and go to a restaurant. And that is what I did—and I felt better emotionally and physically. But I did not know where to go from there. I was in my forties and had never been to a gym, had more weight to lose and didn't know how to build muscle to improve my metabolism.

I searched on Google and found a few gyms in Sacramento, and after contacting a few, decided to go meet Forest. He was great. He was welcoming, not shaming, and confident that I could reach my weight loss goals. I told him I had never lifted a dumbbell before, much less a kettlebell, but that was okay.

After training at FVT for about a year, my weight was in the 120s—I COULD NOT BELIEVE IT! I was so happy both mentally and physically and loved shopping for clothes again (including workout clothes!). I bought a bikini (okay, like ten of them), something I had not done in twenty years! I know it shouldn't really matter, that we do love ourselves for who we are, but, man, it felt good. The next year, my husband and I did our first Spartan Race, a feat I never would have imagined for myself, and I know I would not have done it without the support of Forest.

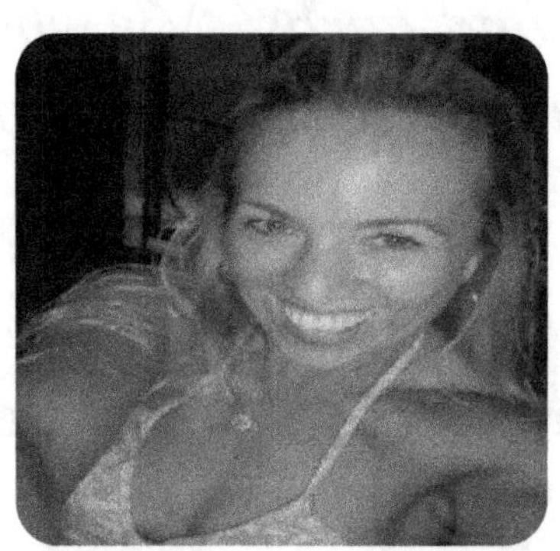

I would say be consistent, don't give up even when life throws you a curveball (or two), and believe that you are worth it, because you are. I am now working on very precise fitness goals—losing fifty plus pounds was hard work for sure, but now I'm attacking my body fat percentage. I feel better, look better, have stopped needing to take blood pressure and cholesterol medications, and have so much more confidence (hello sundress season!). I am so glad I found Forest and his team, who have never wavered in their commitment to my success, even as those goals change over the years."

RUBEN AND JENNY LOST 35+ POUNDS

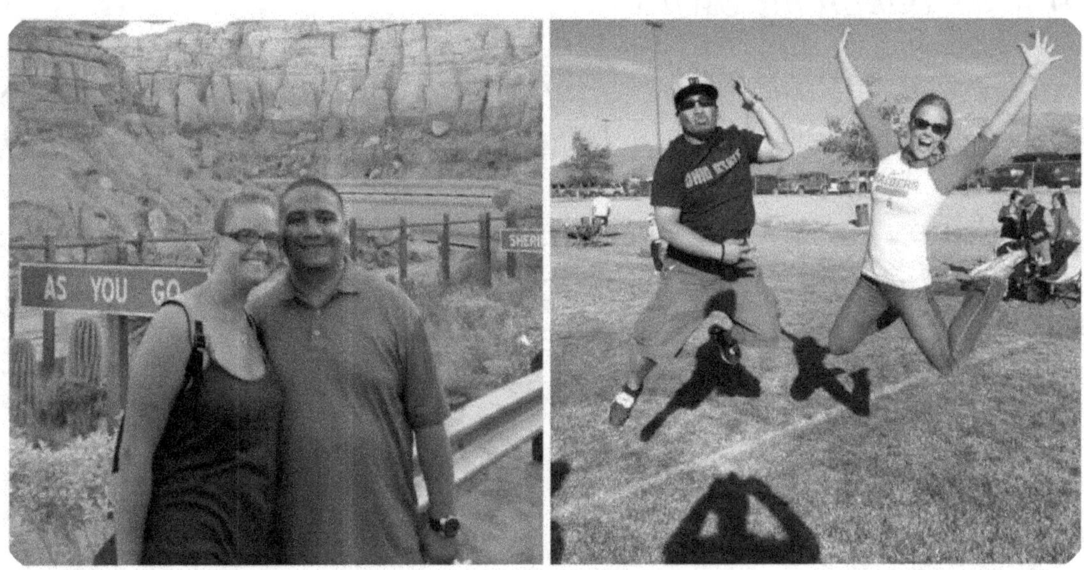

Ruben and Jenny were always very active and involved in sports in their younger days . . . but after college, and especially when they started working full time, fitness was put on the back burner.

They came to me looking for a program they could do together. At the time, they were both tired at the end of their workdays and didn't have much energy.

Ruben was also looking for a workout that he would enjoy, but also wouldn't be intimidating for Jenny.

Ruben said:

"I didn't just want to join a gym where I'd be over by the weights doing bench presses and she'd have to be my spotter or something."

And Jenny said:

"I was apprehensive about working with Forest at first because I hadn't done any sort of strength training before, I had only done cardio.

And I didn't know if it would be worth it to work out here versus just trying to work out on my own.

I was worried about the time commitment. I'm always really busy with teaching, and I wasn't sure how it was going to fit into my schedule."

Ruben and Jenny have been working with me for two and a half years now . . . check out what they have to say about the results that they have experienced:

Jenny:

"We've been working with Forest for two and a half years now, and after that first year I felt like I was in the best shape I've ever been in. My cardio endurance is back up, and I'm stronger than I've ever been. I never would have imagined I'd be doing push-ups and things like that, and now it comes easily to me. It's amazing to see what a huge difference working with Forest has made not only with my strength but also with changes in my body.

I've lost around fifteen pounds from when I first started, but more importantly, I'm leaner, I've gained more muscle, and I've changed my body composition. A lot of people think that I've lost a lot of weight, but it's mostly the change in my body composition that makes me look fitter. And I'm a lot stronger. When I started I was doing overhead presses with eight- to ten-pound dumbbells, and now I'm using twenty-six pounds. I can also do ten toe push-ups in a row, and when I started I couldn't even do one full-range push-up from my knees! There's a huge difference in my upper-body strength."

Ruben:

"I was pretty large and in charge before I started coming here. I've lost about twenty pounds, and I feel really good now. I'm definitely a lot stronger, and I have a lot more endurance. I couldn't do a pull-up when I first started, and now I can do eight to ten."

Overall we've definitely adopted a much healthier, active lifestyle since starting to work with Forest. Not to mention a more positive outlook toward working out and nutrition. It's just been a very positive experience and has definitely transferred into other areas of our lives."

RYAN LOST 20+ POUNDS

Ryan started working with me about a year ago looking to lose weight, shed body fat, and gain back the fitness he once had.

He had been fit and active in the past, but for various reasons, let himself slip out of peak condition.

In the last twelve months, training at the studio three or four times per week and laser-focusing on his nutrition, Ryan has done the following:

- Lost about twenty pounds
- Dropped over 8 percent body fat
- Run a 7:08 mile for the first time since he was eighteen
- Planned for not one but TWO half marathons in the next couple of months

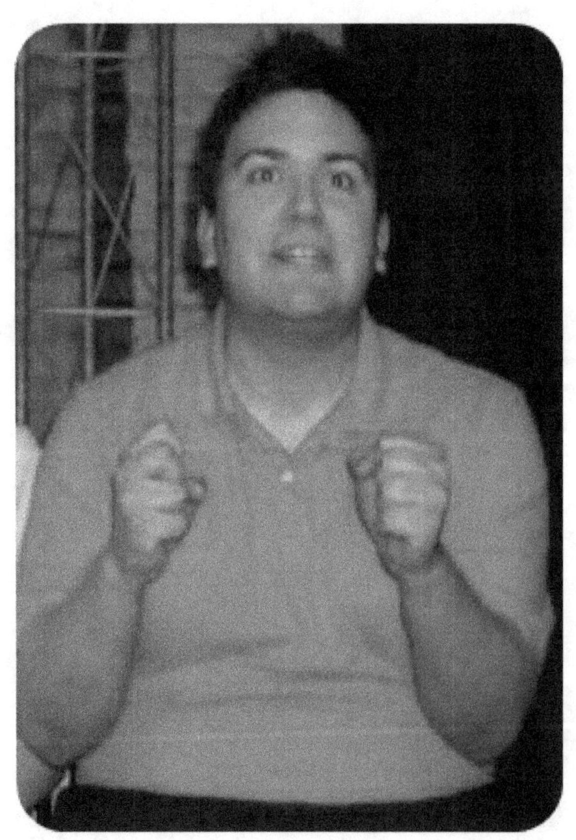

Ryan before working with me:

"The picture here is from January 2010. I weighed 235 pounds, was nearly completely sedentary, and was generally had a terrible physical state and mental outlook. Just a few years before I was the slimmest I'd ever been as an adult, at 185 pounds and regularly exercising, but still with some poor habits. In high school I ran cross-country and track and couldn't keep weight on from the mileage; that all changed once I graduated and stopped the activity and started a terrible spiral of weight gain, probably a mild depression because of it, and a debilitating helplessness in which I never took responsibility or action to be healthier.

At the time this 2010 photo was taken, not yet thirty years old, I was winded walking up the parking garage stairs to my car, and perpetually buying larger and larger clothes. One day in January, I read about a person in the Capitol community who'd died at just forty, quite unexpectedly. That day, after another struggle up the stairs and seeing this picture, I decided to make a change.

I began exercising again, logging my food into an app on my phone, and within a few months I'd lost almost twenty-five lbs. Going at it solo with no structure proved extremely challenging after a while, and by late 2012 I'd gained back about half the weight. All the while, I'd watched Erik transform himself through diet and exercise and thought, "What is stopping me? Why don't I make that change?"

One year ago today, I walked into Forest Vance Training Inc. for a 6:00 a.m. boot camp, late, having eaten hardly anything, and terrified about the physical demands of the workout. After nearly passing out more than once, I gritted through it and quite literally could barely walk up my own stairs at home from the intensity of that first workout on my previously fit body, which was in such desperate need of rehabilitation. I hurt for days, even after my second session and my third. I could barely change my clothes during the final performances of the show I was doing that weekend, but despite that hurt I felt good."

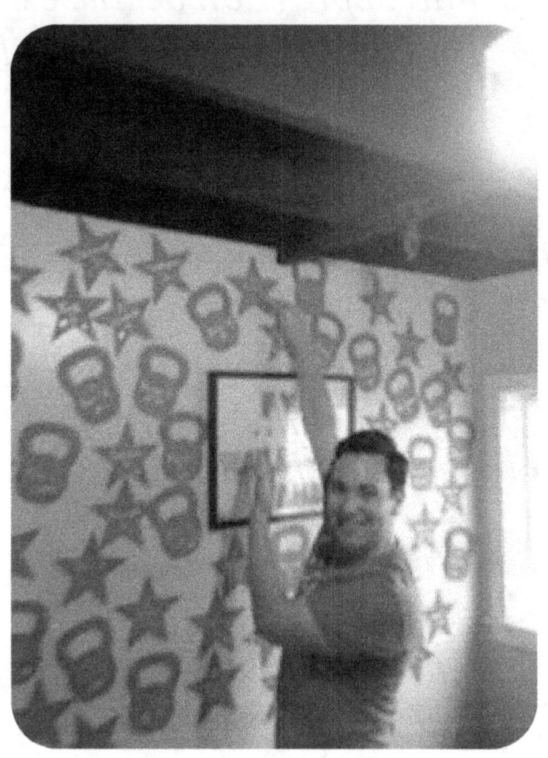

Last February I weighed 222 pounds and was nearly 28 percent body fat. Today I weigh 205 pounds and am 19.8 percent body fat—below 20 percent for the first time since I was a teenager, probably. Today I'm a few weeks away from my first half marathon. Two weeks ago I ran a mile in 7:08 for the first time since I was eighteen. Today I'm planning for my second half marathon.

My reason why isn't just one reason: there are many. I joined FVT as a client because I don't want to die of something preventable at age forty, because I don't want to make excuses about why I can't do something, because I want to challenge myself to do things I didn't think I could do. My reason why is because I didn't want to be on heartburn medicine for the rest of my life, or keep buying pants in larger sizes, or wheeze on the way up the stairs to my car.

My reason is not to be thin or lose weight—though that was part of my goal, it is no longer the most important one. My reason is that I want to look in the mirror and see a healthy person who goes outside and enjoys the weather, enjoys a run, enjoys how exercise and good choices make me feel, and know that living healthy isn't about a diet or the next six months . . . it's about living a whole life. That's my reason why.

PART 2:

THE CORE KETTLEBELL CHALLENGE

"If you are distressed by anything external, the pain is not due to the thing itself, but to your estimate of it; and this you have the power to revoke at any moment."

—*Marcus Aurelius,* **Meditations**

FOUNDATIONS WEEK

When we get new personal training clients at FVT, one of our primary goals is to get them up to speed on their kettlebell form as fast as possible.

It's always form and technique BEFORE we stack on the intensity.

This sets us up for long-term success.

This is why BEFORE you start the "official" CORE Kettlebell program, you're going to do a "Foundations" week.

It's kind of like a kettlebell and bodyweight workshop—where you'd come to my studio and we would work on form and drills to improve and more—but it's split up over a one-week period.

Adequate strength and proper movement are required to do all the exercises. If you are coming in weak and/or tight and/or inflexible, understand that it will take a little time - and that's okay. I want you to practice each of the exercises in this section until you feel comfortable with safe and effective form. If you need to continue to repeat this week— for two weeks, three weeks, four weeks—**you can do it for up to twelve weeks before moving on to the main program**. It is critical that THIS comes BEFORE adding intensity—to avoid injury, and for maximum results.

<u>YOUR SELF-ASSESSMENT</u>

The other great thing is that as you go through these movements slowly and deliberately with practice, you'll get sort of a "self-assessment"— you can see where you are tight and where you need to work on strength and mobility, etc.

Fortunately, I have kept the program simple (NOT easy, but simple). There are just a few basic movements you will need to learn. These movements, and small variations of them, will get you through the full six-week program.

Day One (Monday)

1) Hip Hinge (technique drill): do 2 sets, 5 reps each, rest 30 seconds between

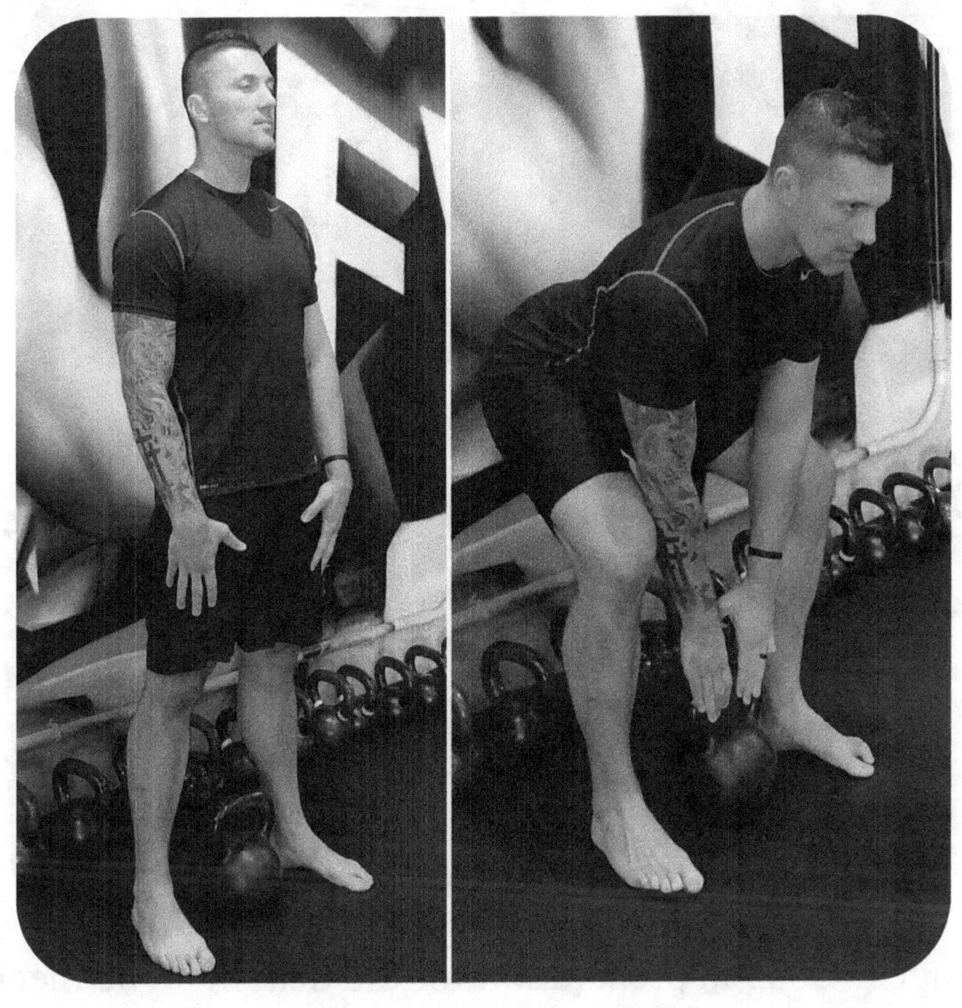

Start standing facing away from a wall, with your heels eighteen to twenty-four inches away. Initiate the move by pushing your butt back toward the wall. Stop when your hands touch the kettlebell. Note that your spine should be neutral, your hips should be higher than your knees, and your shoulders should be higher than your hips.

2) Deadlift (technique drill): 2 sets, 5 reps each, rest 30 seconds between

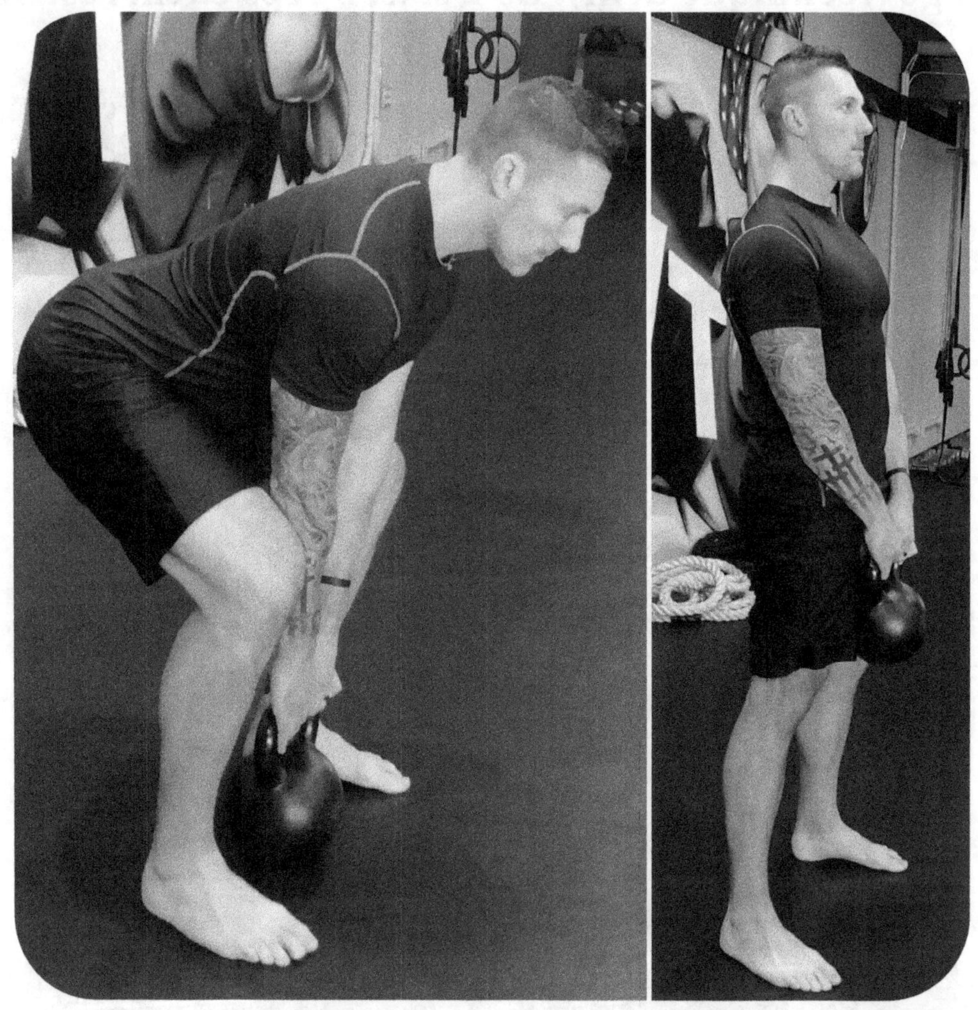

The hip hinge is done in preparation for the deadlift. The mechanics are the same, except now, you pick up the kettlebell. Note that the body is in a straight line—from the ankles to the knees to the hips to the shoulders to the neck—at the top/completion of the exercise.

3) Swing: 2 sets, 10 reps each, rest 30 seconds between

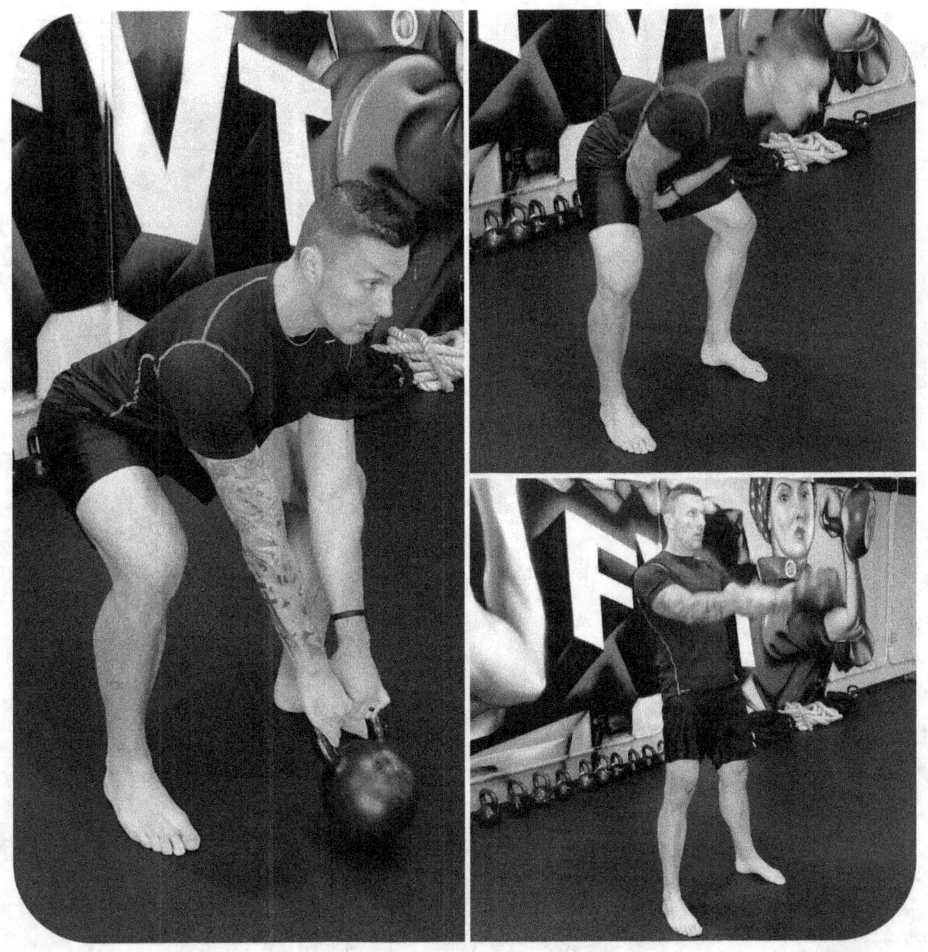

Stand with feet shoulder width (or slightly wider) apart. Assume the starting position with the kettlebell approximately eighteen to twenty-four inches in front of the feet, hips down and back (but above the knees), shoulders back, chest up, and in a neutral spine position. Swing the kettlebell back between the legs, keeping the handle above the knee level. The kettlebell will swing up to chest level or slightly higher, but will stay below the eyes. Repeat for desired number of reps, and return to starting position in the same way the movement began.

4) One-arm swing: 2 sets, 5 reps per side, rest 30 seconds between

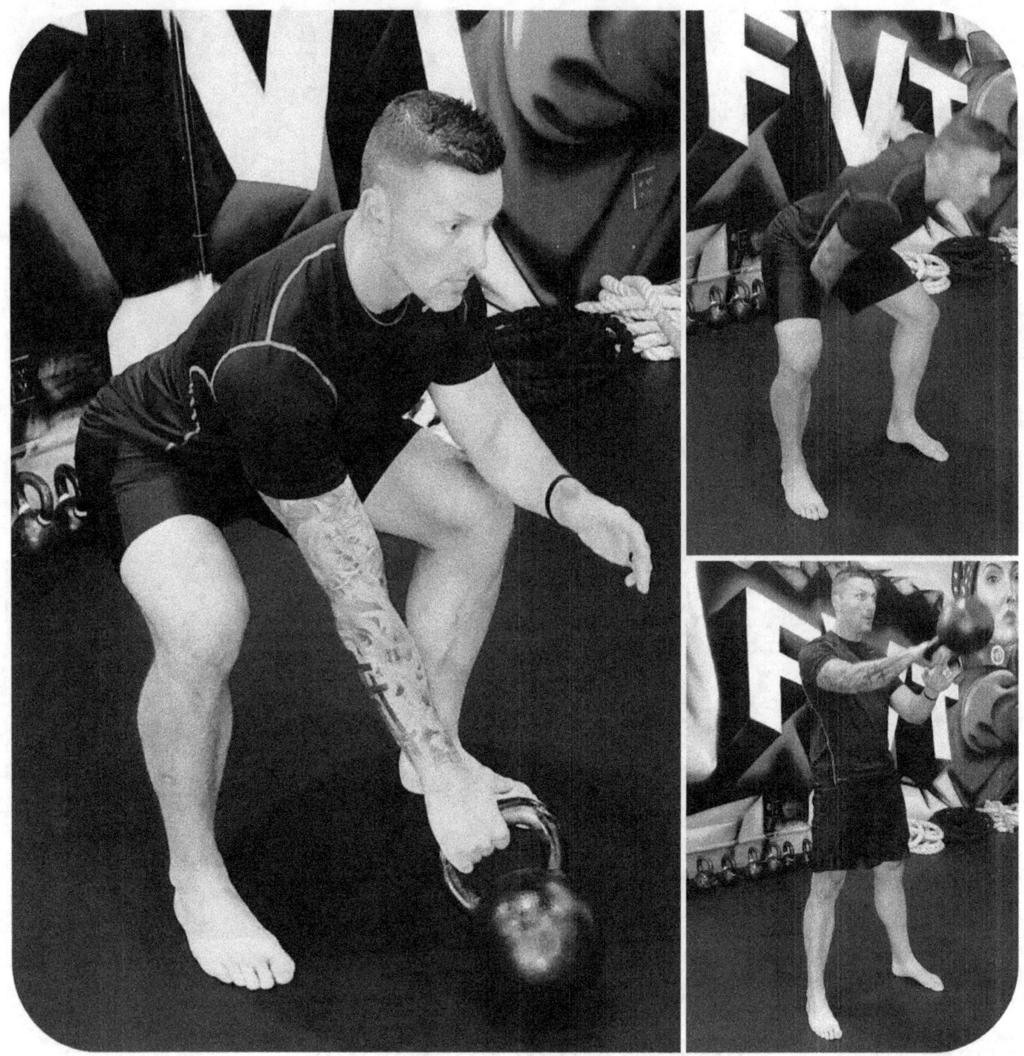

The one-arm swing is like the two-hand swing—we just have one hand on the kettlebell. Think of the one-arm swing as an anti-rotational exercise. The shoulders and body should stay square. The core should stay tight.

5) "Finisher" workout:

Set your timer to go off at 30 second intervals. For the first 30 second interval, do kettlebell swings. These can be with one or two hands, your choice. For the second 30 second interval, do 30 seconds of active recovery (see options below). Repeat this sequence a total of six times, for a total of six sets of swings and six sets of active recovery.

Active recovery options:

Run in Place

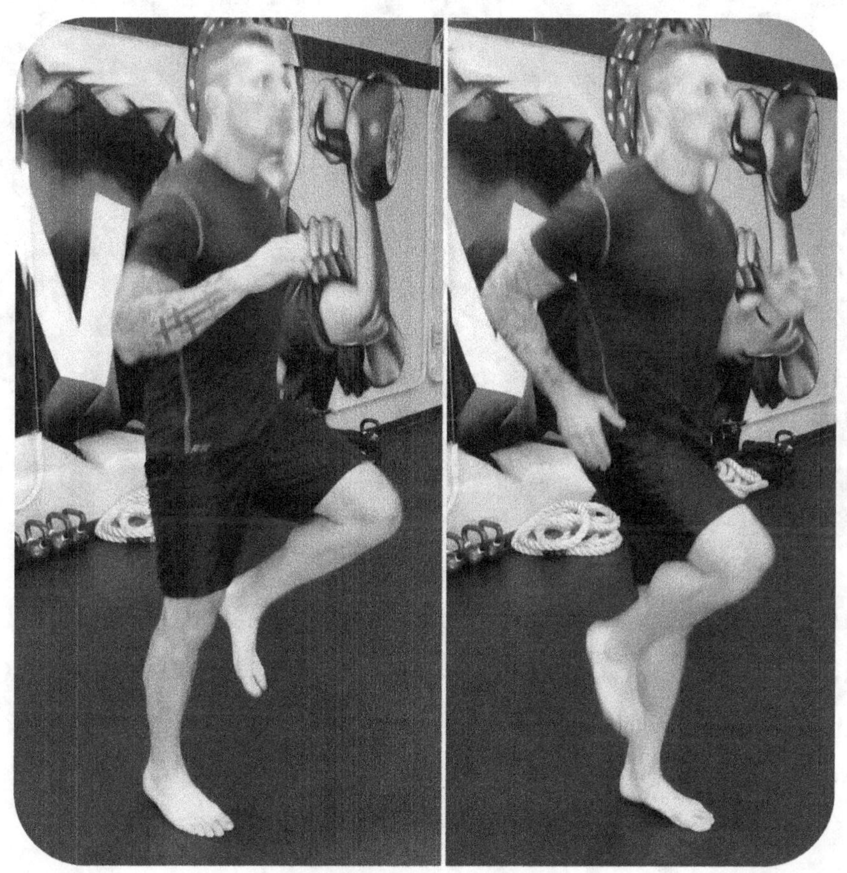

Pick your knees up and run on the spot. Try to get some good arm action to power your lower body. You can bring your knees as low or as high as you want to adjust the intensity level.

Jumping Jacks

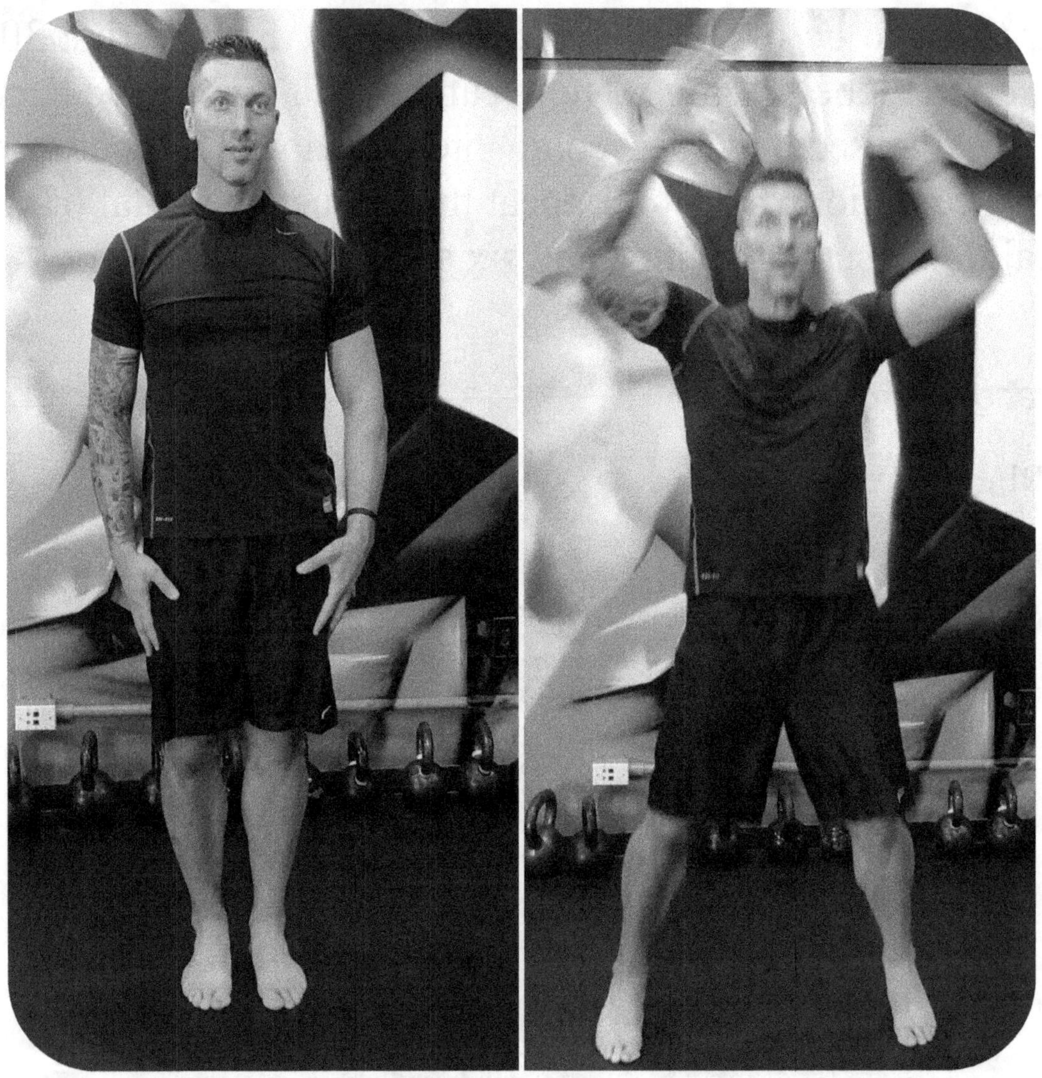

Start standing tall with your arms at your sides. Jump your legs apart to about shoulder width while at the same time bringing your hands up over your head. Jump your feet back in and bring your hands back down to starting position. That's one rep.

Day Two (Tuesday)

1) Kettlebell Squats: 2 sets, 10 reps each, rest 30 seconds between

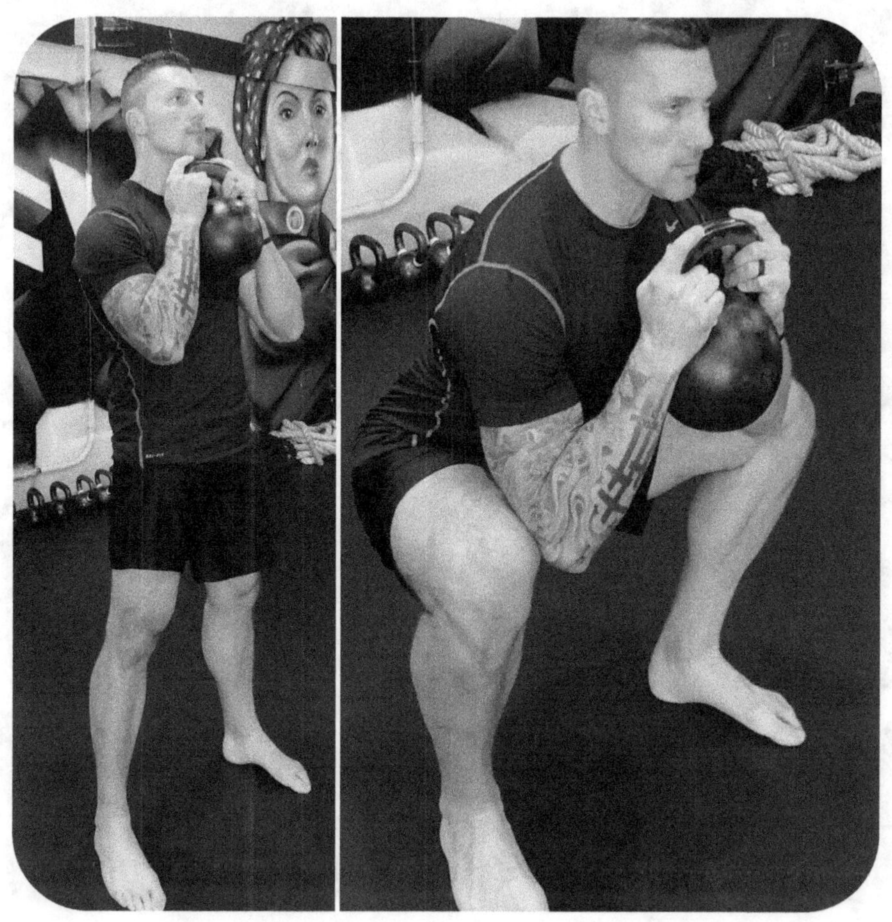

Pick a kettlebell up off of the floor with one smooth motion to get into starting the starting position pictured above. When you pick up the kettlebell, maintain a neutral spine. Stand with feet shoulder width apart. Lower hips back and down to start the movement. Hips will descend lower than the knees at the bottom. The lumbar curve is maintained, and the heels stay down on the ground. The knees stay in line with the toes. The top of the movement is completed with full knee and hip extension. The kettlebell is placed on the ground in the same fashion that it was picked up.

2) Lunges: 2 sets, 5 reps each leg, rest 30 seconds between

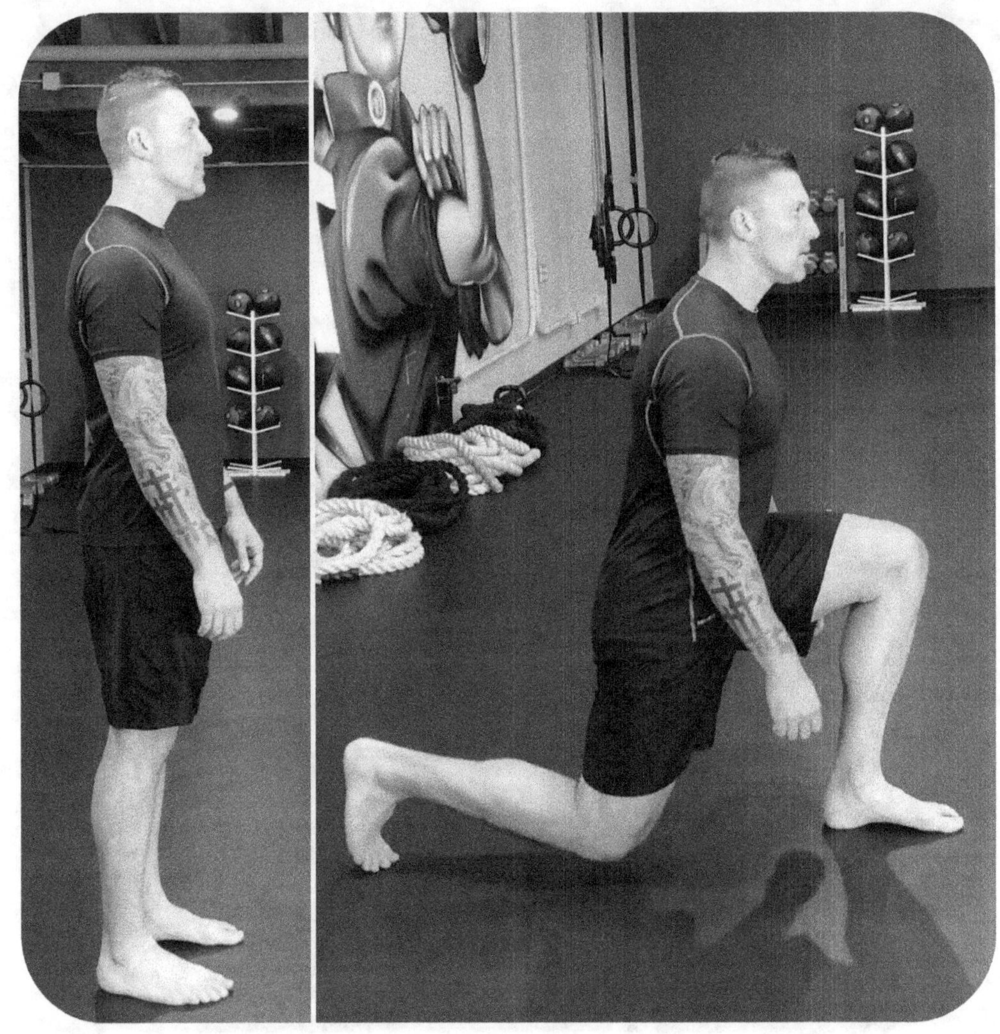

Start in a standing position with the feet together, standing tall, with the chest up and shoulders down and back. One leg steps forward. Keep heel of the forward leg down. Lower the torso until the back knee touches the ground. The forward shin stays relatively vertical. The movement is complete at full hip and knee extension. The opposite leg begins the next step.

3) Plank hold: 2 sets, 30-second holds, rest 30 seconds between.

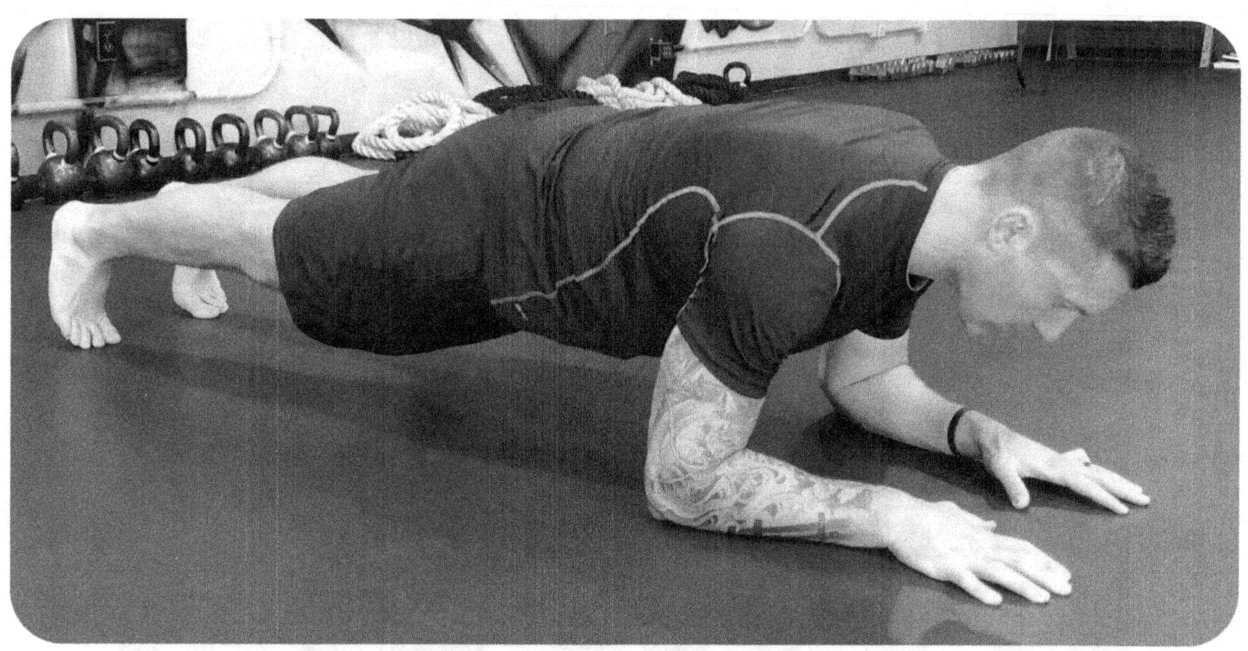

Assume plank position. Both forearms are in contact with the ground. Eyes are focused between the hands. Lower back/hips are in a neutral position. Legs are locked and feet are together.

4) Push up: 2 sets, 10 reps, rest 30 seconds between

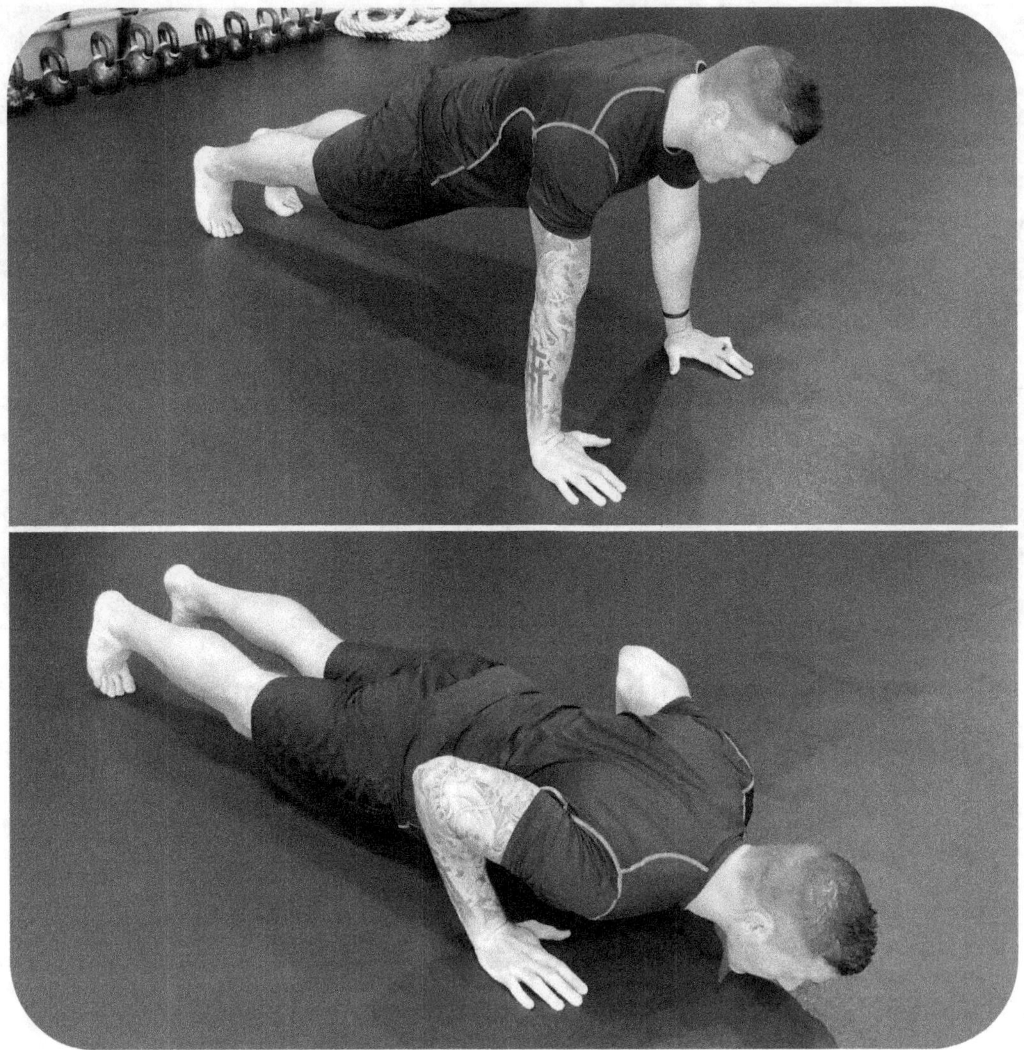

Hands are on the ground, shoulder width apart. Legs are straight, with only the balls of the feet on the ground (men – toe push-up) OR body is straight, with only the knees and hands on the ground. Begin the movement with the arms extended. Lower the chest and thighs to the ground. The body remains rigid. The elbows move closer to the hips than shoulders. The movement is complete at full arm extension. Holding for one second at the top, candidate will lower their body toward the floor (knees for women, toes for men), breaking at least ninety degrees at the elbow and forearm.

5) Recline Row: 2 sets, 10 reps each, rest 30 seconds between

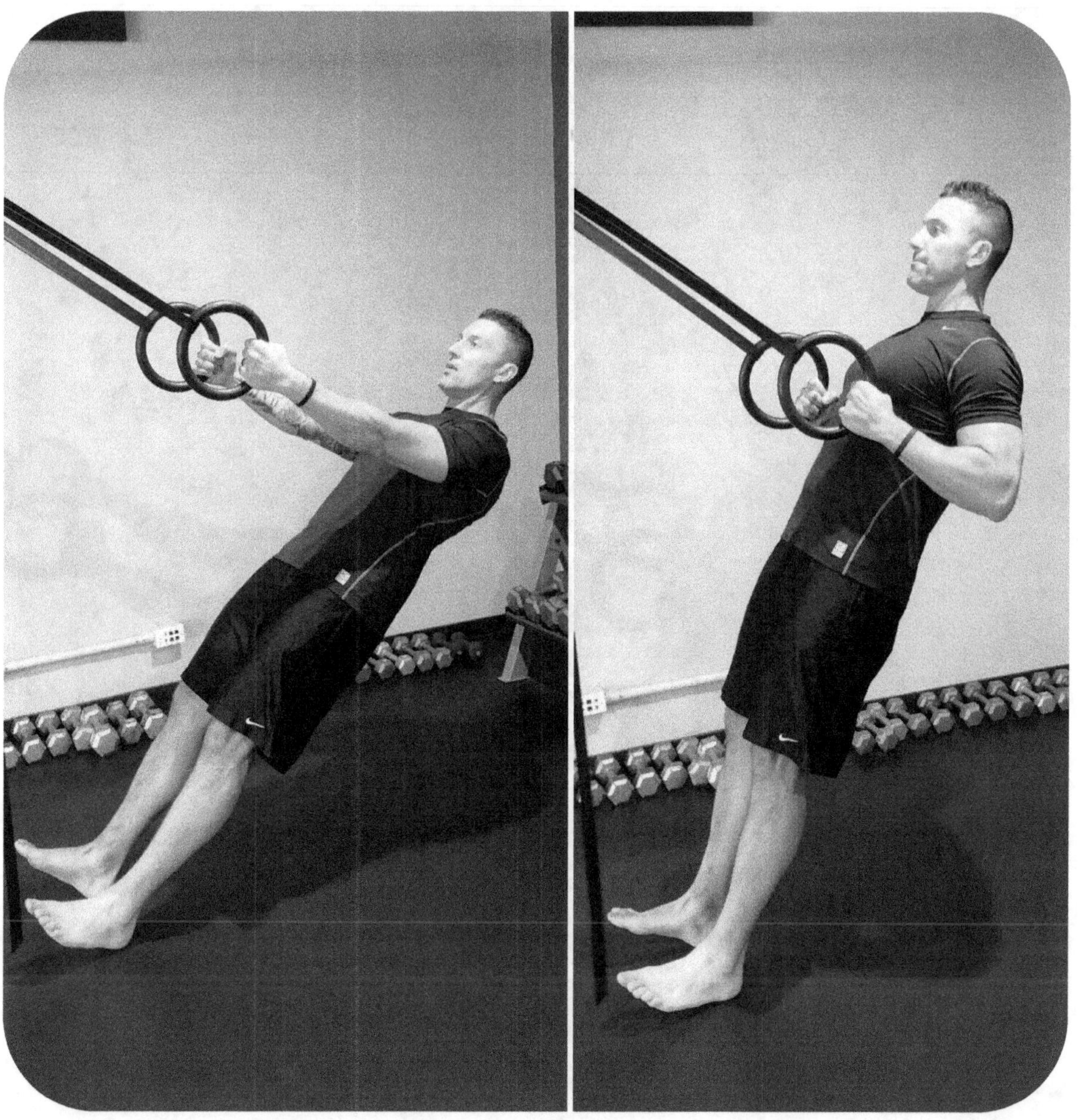

Assume a starting position lying on the ground, directly underneath the point gymnastics rings or a suspension trainer is affixed. Knees are at a ninety-degree angle, and arms are fully extended. Pull yourself toward the rings or suspension trainer until your hands touch the torso, keeping the wrists straight.

6) Pull-Ups: 2 sets, 3 reps, rest 30 seconds between

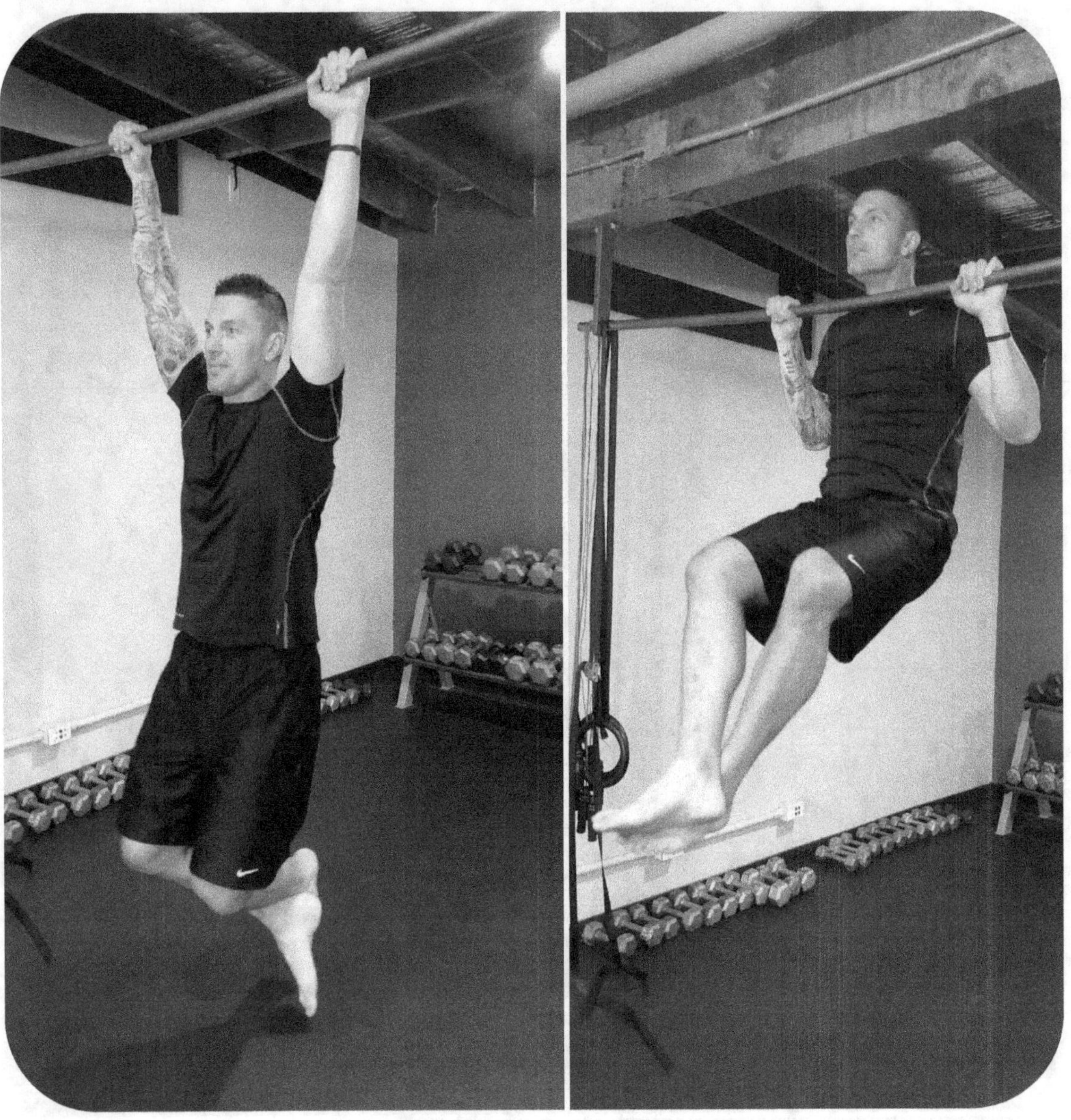

Pull-ups are done with an overhand grip. Start out fully hanging from the bar, with arms fully extended. Pull yourself up, clearing the bar with the chin and cleanly touching the neck or chest at the top. Slowly lower yourself down, under control, until arms are fully extended at the bottom.

7) "Finisher" workout:

- 1 Push-Up (beginner) or 1 Pull-Up (advanced)
- 2 Recline Rows (beginner) or 2 Push-Ups (advanced)
- 3 Bodyweight Squats

followed by

- 2 Push-Ups (beginner) or 2 Pull-Ups (advanced)
- 4 Recline Rows (beginner) or 4 Push-Ups (advanced)
- 6 Bodyweight Squats

. . . continue the pattern (increasing Push-Ups/Pull-Ups by 1 rep, Recline Rows/Pull-Ups by 2, and Squats by 3) until you get to 7 Push-Ups, 14 Recline Rows, and 21 Squats. Rest as needed between exercises and sets.

Day Three (Thursday)

1) Grip/Rack (technique drill): hold for 20 seconds each side; repeat total of 2 times each side

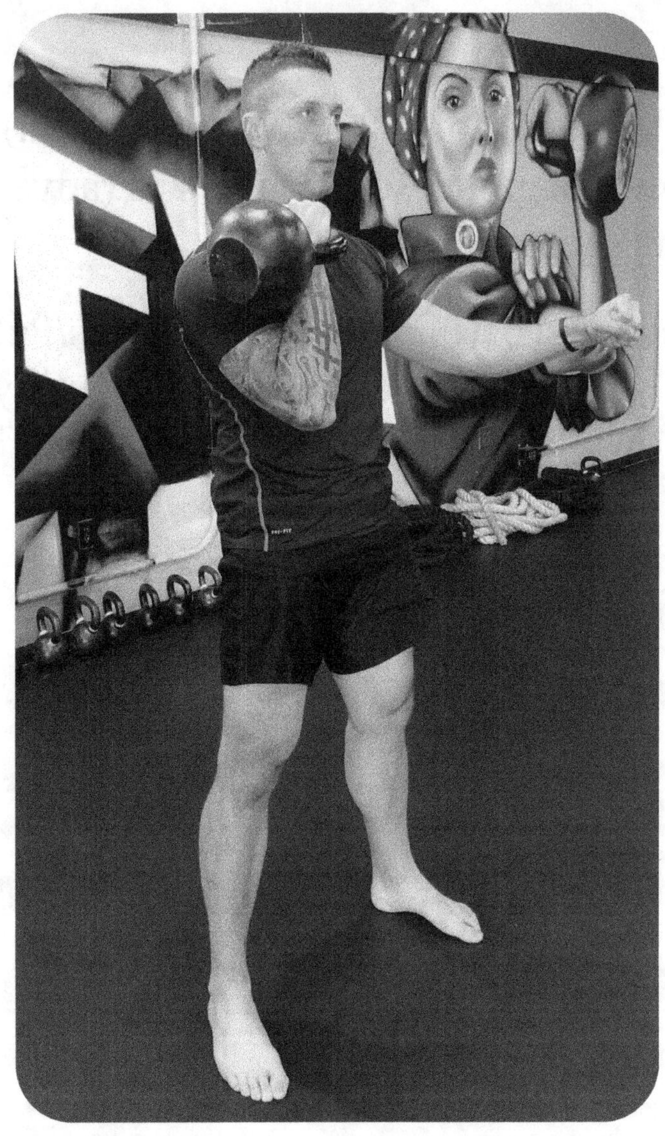

Pick up the kettlebell. Get into the "rack" position: Your forearm should be vertical. Your wrist should be straight. You should be able to touch your collar bone with your thumb. This is the position from which all your pressing and other moves will start—so get comfortable in it.

2) Clean from top down (technique drill): 2 sets, 5 reps each, rest 30 seconds between

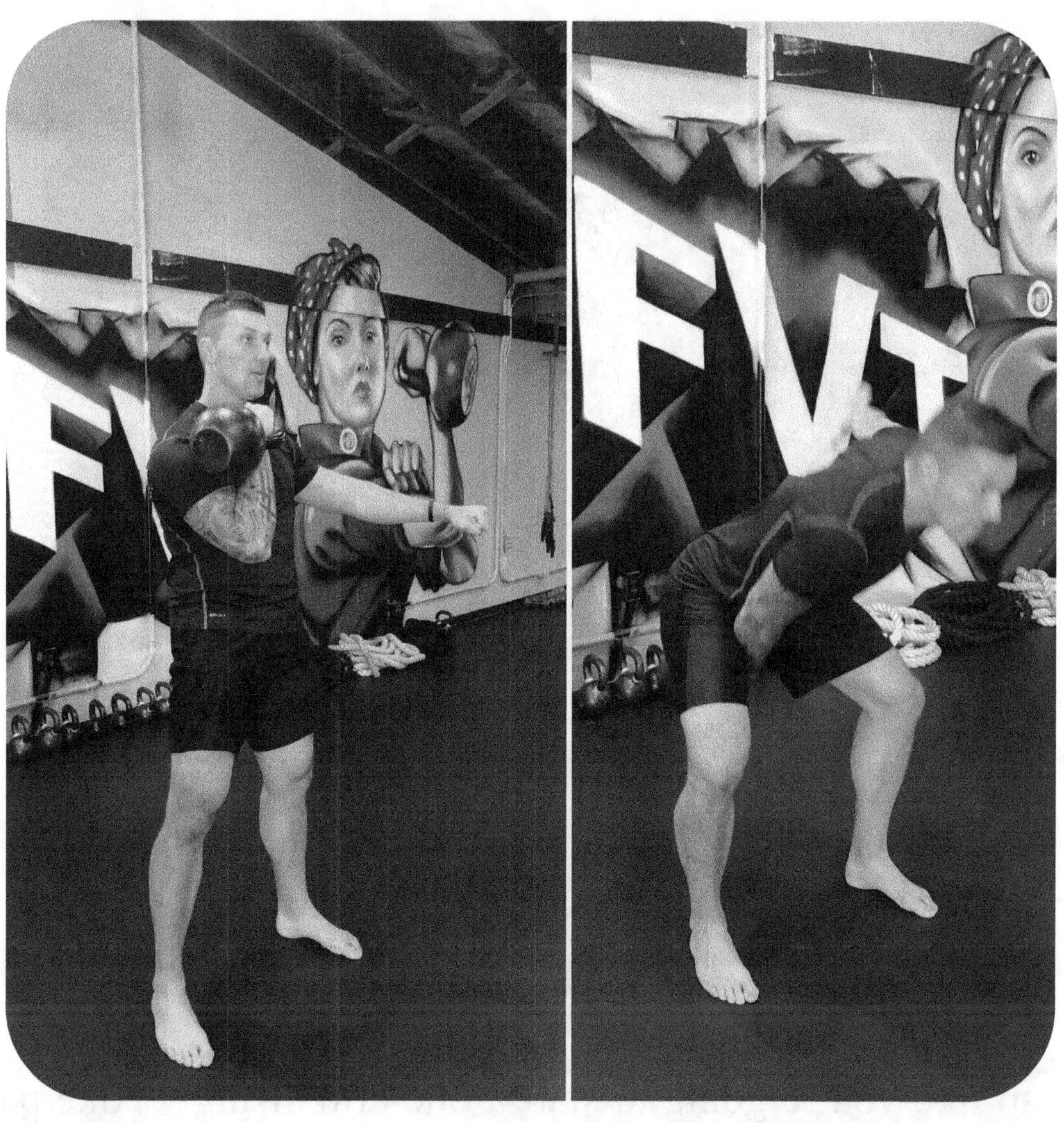

Start in the kettlebell rack position. Drop the kettlebell back between the legs. Try to imagine you are dropping the kettlebell back behind you— but don't actually do it :) Reverse the motion and bring the kettlebell back up to the rack position.

3) Clean from ground (technique drill): 2 sets, 5 reps each, rest 30 seconds between

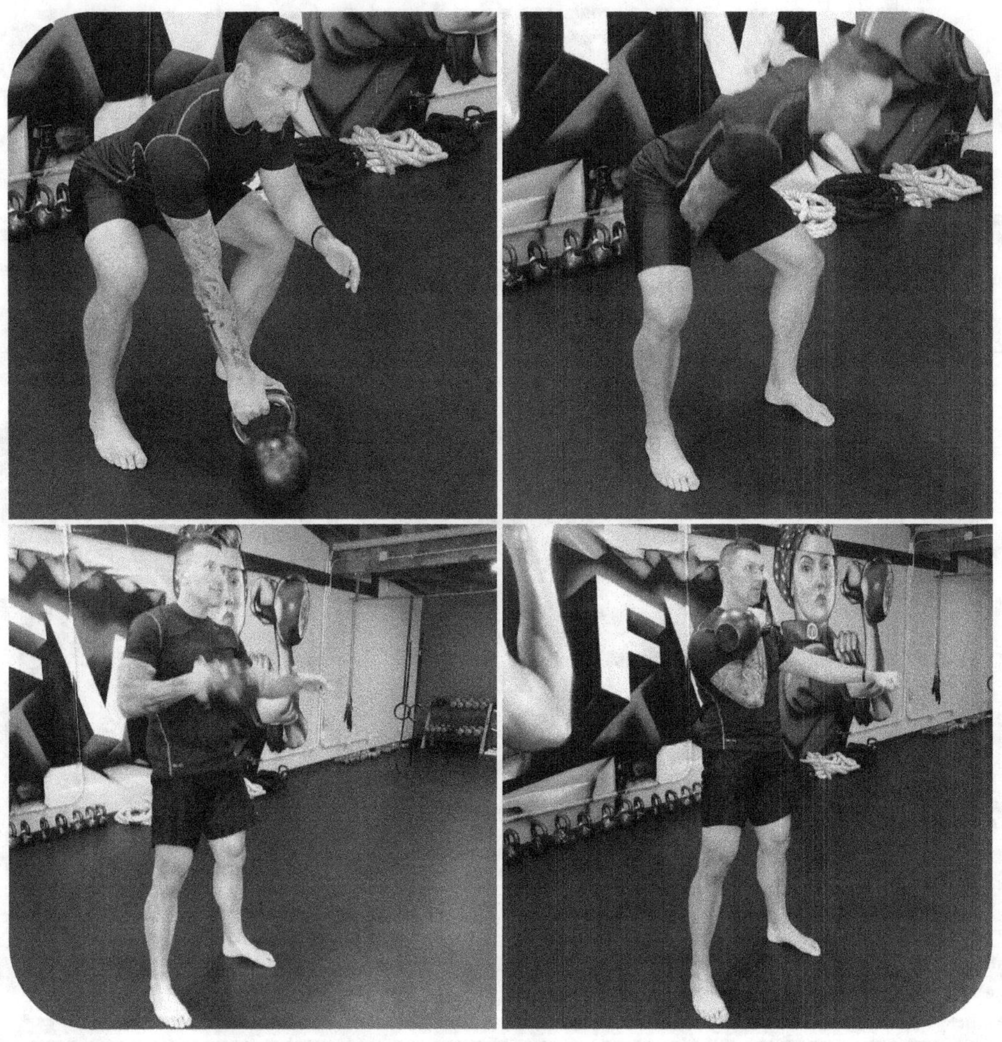

Get set up like you're going to start a one-arm swing. "Hike pass" the kettlebell back through the center of your legs, like a center hiking a football to a quarterback, but then clean it to the shoulder. Same mechanics we've been working on, but now you're starting from the ground. End up with the kettlebell in the rack position at the shoulder. Repeat for reps without putting the kettlebell back on the ground, then return to the ground at the end of the set.

4) "Top down" press (technique drill): 2 sets, 5 reps each, rest 30 seconds between

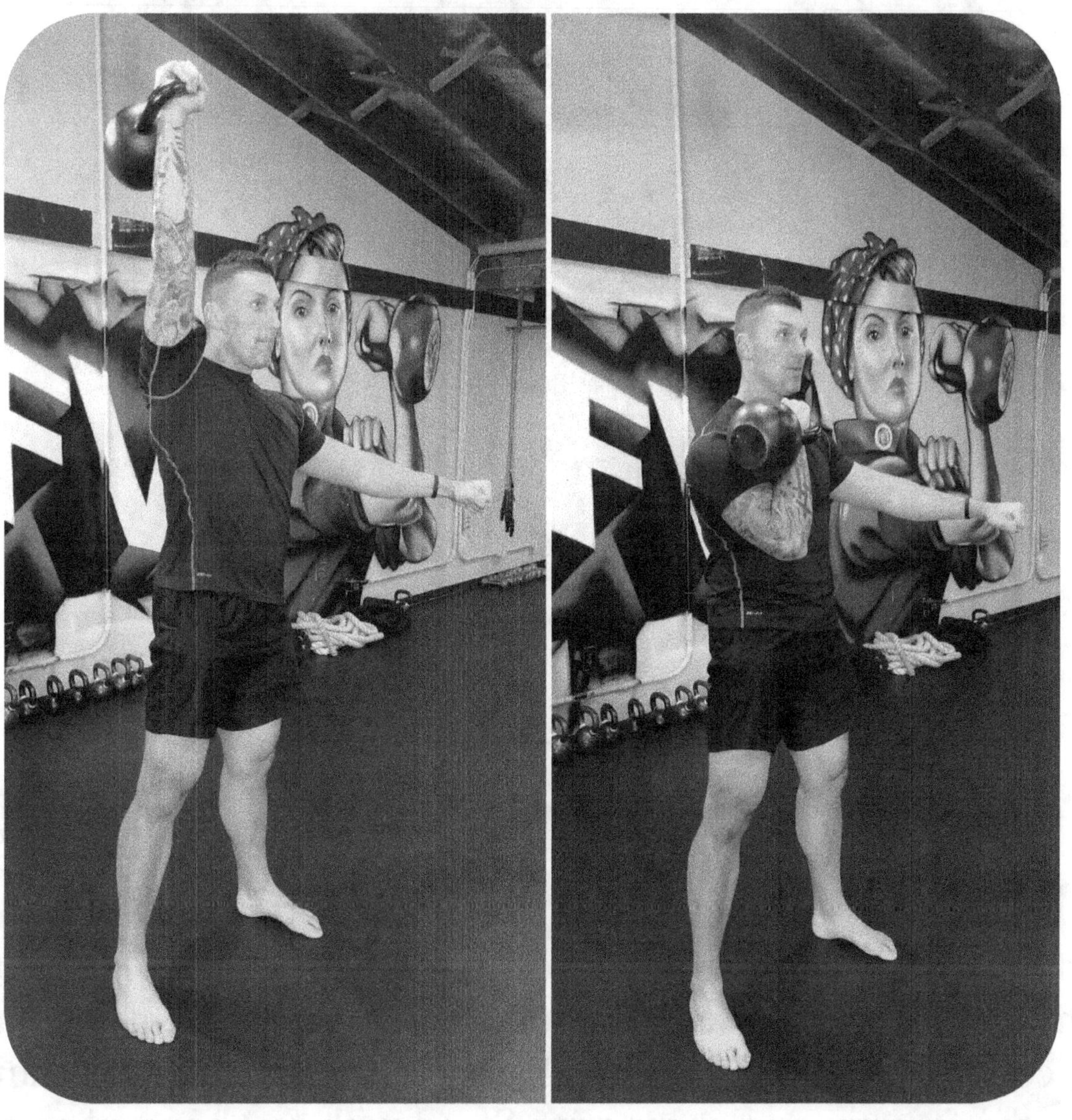

This is like a kettlebell press, but in reverse. Start at the top of the movement, and be active about "pulling" the kettlebell down to the shoulder. Get the groove of the movement. Reverse it and press it back up.

5) Clean and press: 2 sets, 5 reps each, rest 30 seconds between

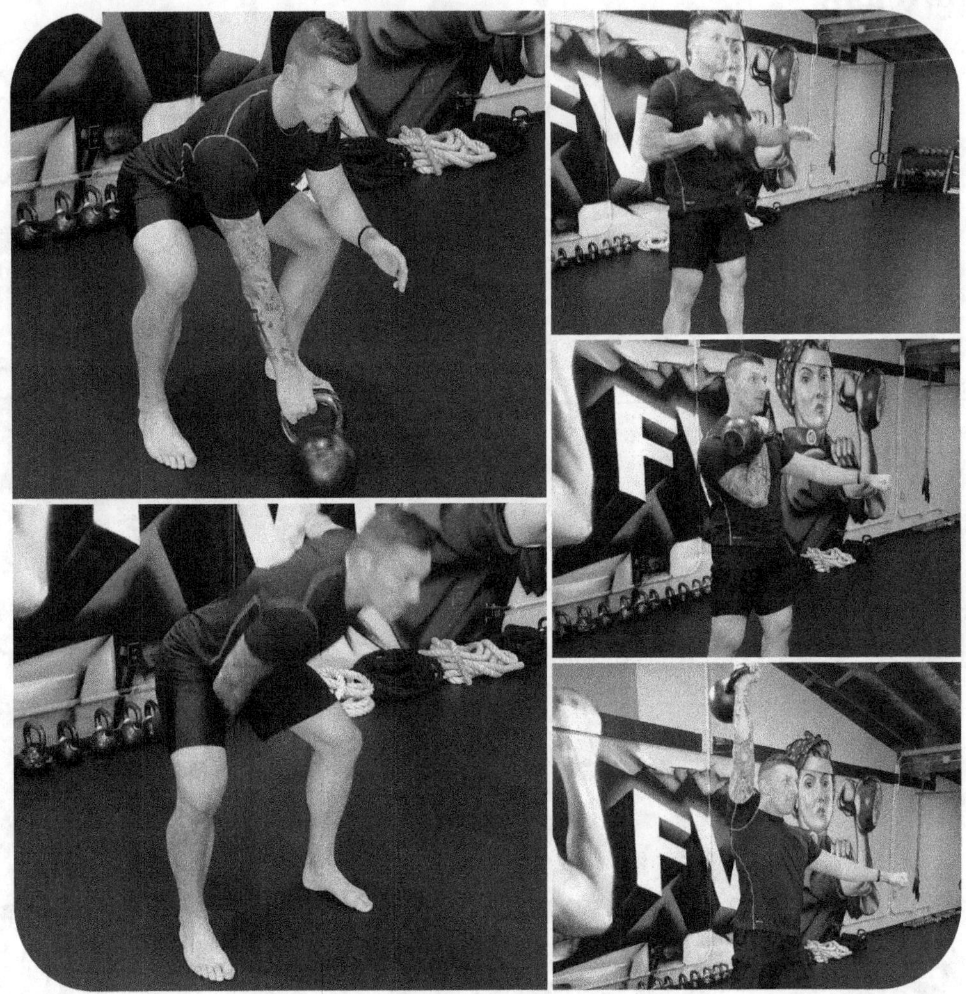

Get into the starting position by cleaning the kettlebell to the shoulder. Assume a rack position with the kettlebell so you can touch the thumb to the collar bone and so the kettlebell is in contact with two additional points, the forearm and upper arm. Stand with feet approximately hip width apart. The elbow will stay underneath the kettlebell as the weight is pressed overhead. The torso and legs stay static during the entire movement. The heels stay down during the entire movement. The movement is complete at full arm extension. The kettlebell is returned to the ground in the same fashion it was picked up.

6) Burpees: 2 sets, 5 reps each, rest 30 seconds between

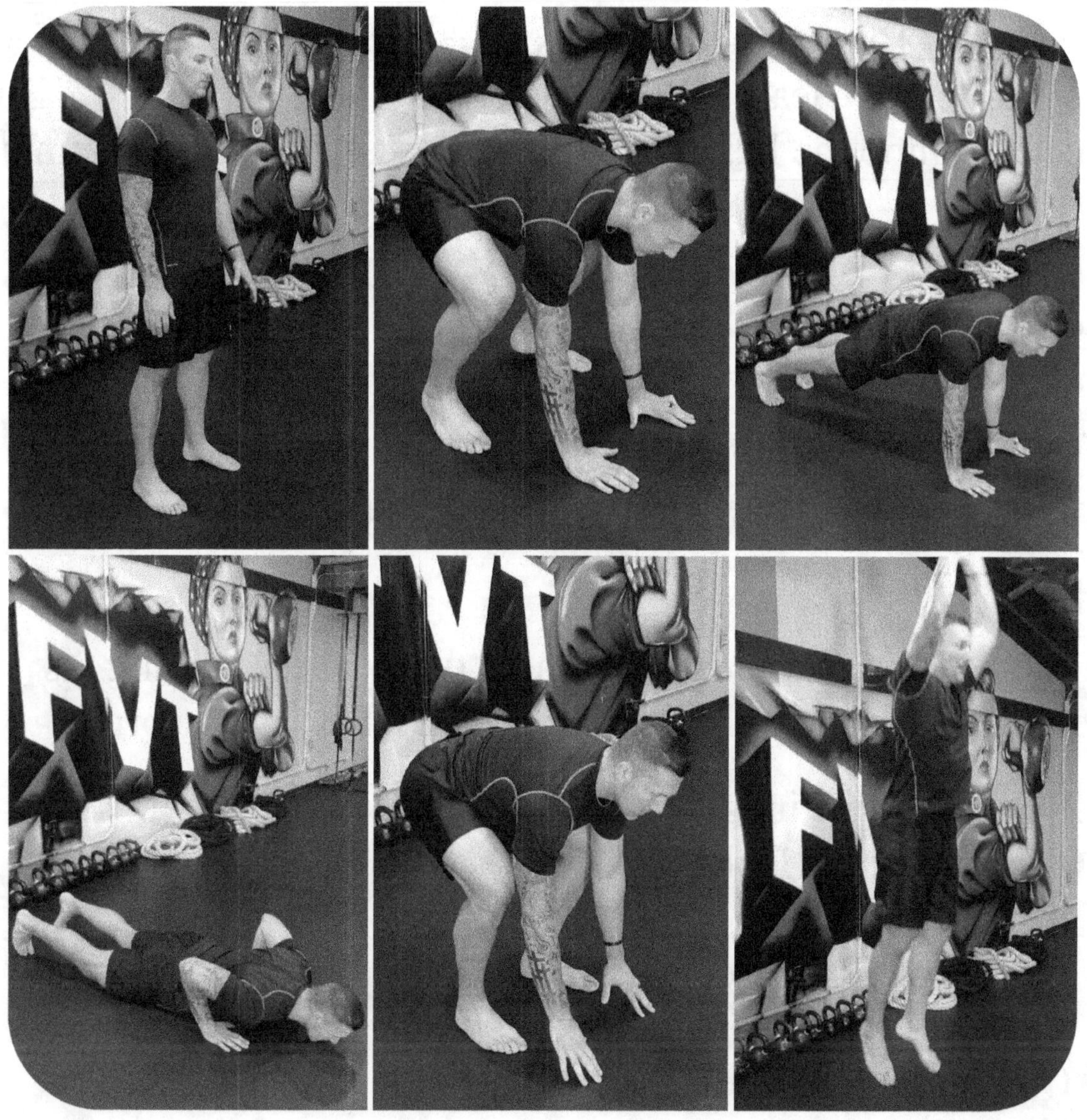

Thighs and torso must touch the ground at the bottom of the movement. Full extension of the body—knees, hips, and upper body—as well as a jump and clap of the hands over the head must be completed at the top of each rep.

7) "Finisher" workout:

Clean + Press / Burpee ladder: 1 Clean + Press right + 1 Clean + Press left + 1 Burpee; 2 Clean + Press right + 2 Clean + Press + 2 Burpees; continue to "climb the ladder" / get as high as you can in 5 minutes.

Day Four (Saturday)

Today, we're putting it all together!

We're taking all the exercises we've learned, and we are going to put them together in a giant circuit.

Go through the following sequence two times, resting as needed between moves, and emphasizing PRACTICE of great form:

- 12 Kettlebell Swings
- 30-second Plank Hold
- 8 Kettlebell Squats
- 5 Pull-Ups OR 12 Recline Rows
- 5 Burpees
- 6 One-Hand Kettlebell Swings (per side)
- 8 Push-Ups
- 6 Lunges (per side)
- 5 Pull-Ups OR 12 Recline Rows
- 5 Burpees

<u>One-Arm Kettlebell Row – Bonus Move</u>

Here is an extra exercise that we did not cover in the Foundations week section, but that we will use in the main workout section. Practice this move and learn the technique before starting the Challenge. See how to do it below:

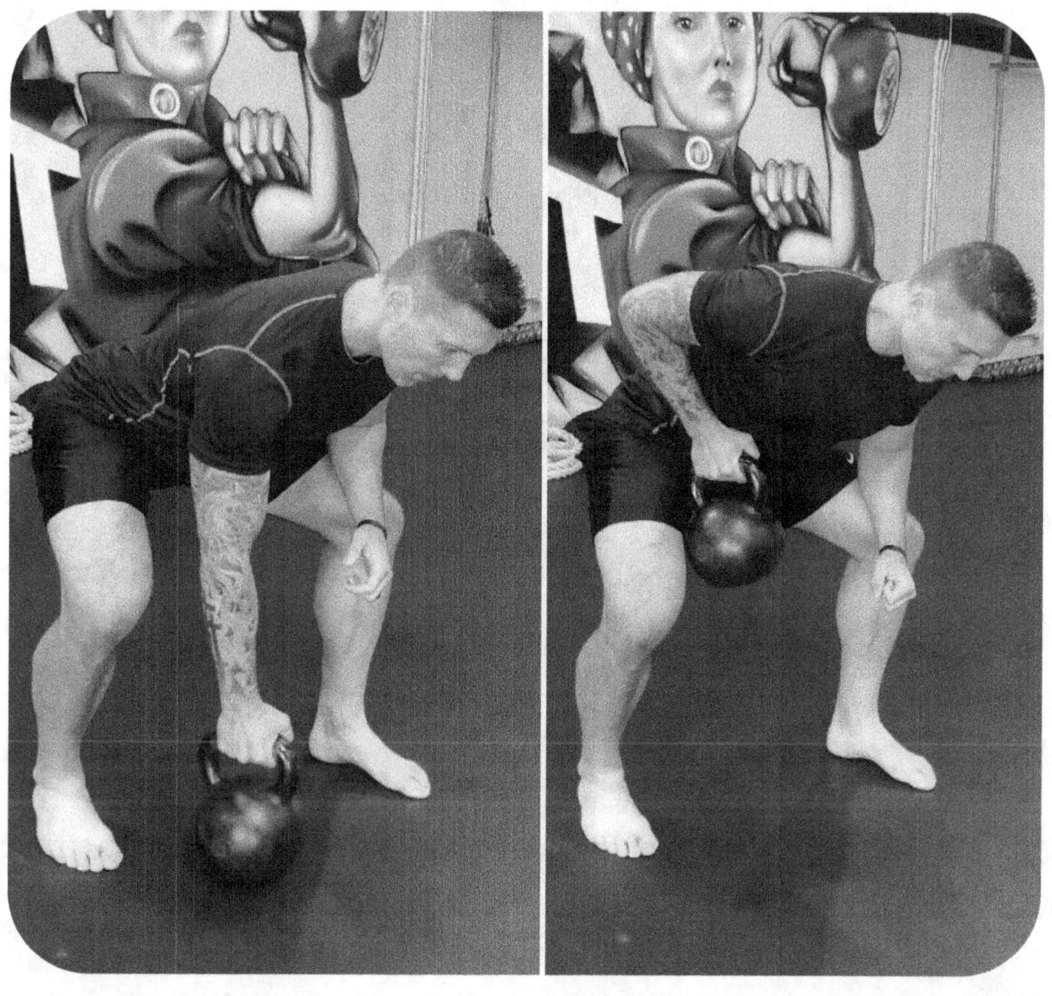

Start by using your body as the bench. The kettlebell is placed to the side of the front foot to start. The knee of the front foot is kept in alignment with the toe. The front forearm is resting on the front thigh. The back leg is grounded and stable. Start the movement by pulling the kettlebell to the torso—approximately belly button level. The spine stays in a neutral position.

TEST IN – PERFORMANCE TESTING

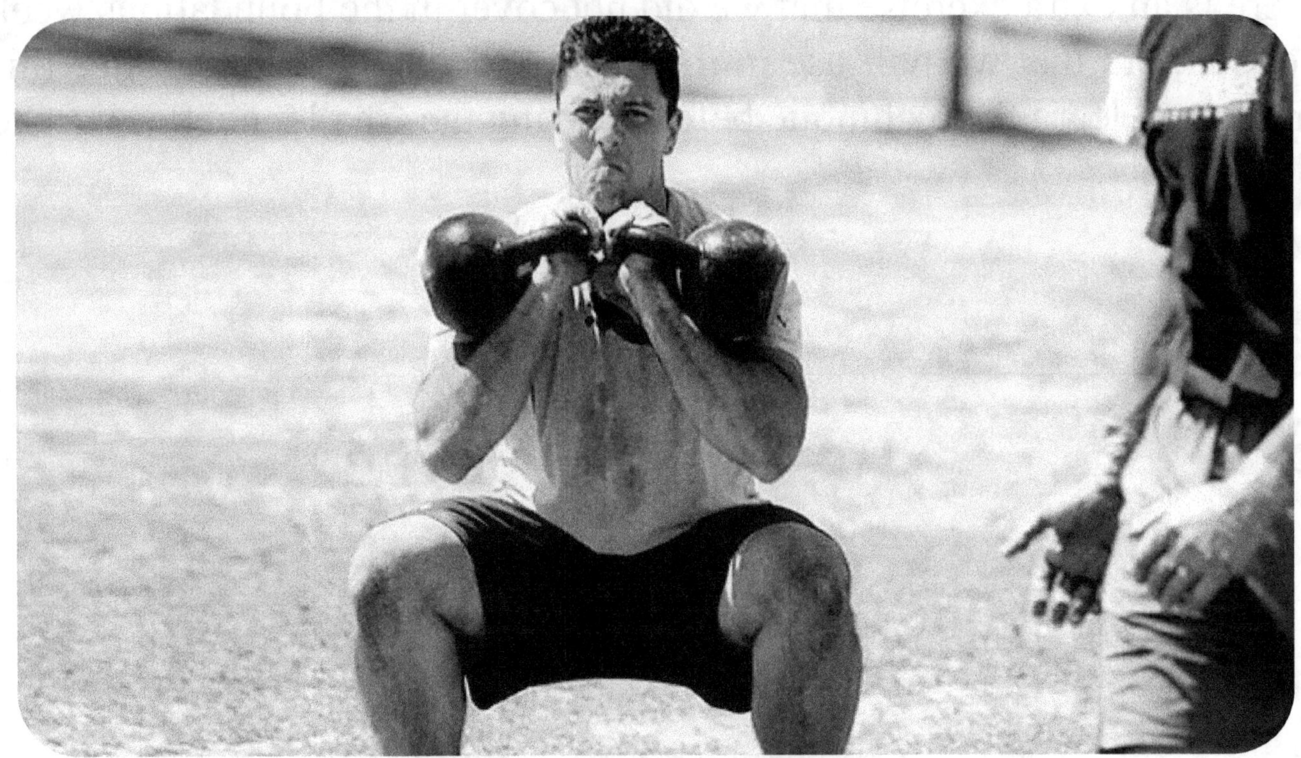

Now we're officially ready to start the 40-day program!

But before we begin, we need to test in.

Because <u>C</u>hallenge-<u>O</u>riented, <u>R</u>esults-<u>E</u>arned is what the CORE Kettlebell Challenge is all about.

You see, when I was playing college football, we always did performance testing at the end of winter and the end of summer.

These were the two periods of the year where we were really focused on lifting and conditioning.

We'd max out bench press, squat, and power cleans, as well as testing things like the 40-yard dash and the vertical jump.

I always looked forward to these tests—which might not be a surprise by now if you're getting to know me—because they gave me a great idea of where I was starting and how all the hard work I put in had paid off.

These also happened to be the times of year when I tended to be in the best physical shape and have the lowest body fat percentage.

So the performance tests in the CORE Kettlebell Challenge are based around these same concepts.

We have you test in at the beginning, do a mid-Challenge test, and test out at the end.

We are going for quantifiable performance results—which in turn will help you lose fat, gain lean muscle, and get in top-notch condition.

I want you to do these tests at the following times:

- At the start of the program—on day 1
- Midway through the program—on day 20
- At the end of the program—on day 40

This will allow you to see your progress.

And remember, go at your own pace. If you have not worked out for a while, do NOT overdo it. Do what your body can do. We are using this as a way to see improvement over the course of the program.

1 – One-Hand Kettlebell Swings

Set clock for thirty-second intervals. Starting at the beginning of each interval, perform ten reps of one-hand swings on each side (alternating hands each set). After finishing one rep, rest for the time interval between that rep and when the next thirty-second interval starts. Repeat for a total of ten rounds, alternating hands each set. (You'll do five sets of ten reps per side).

Use the heaviest weight you can while completing all 100 reps with perfect form. Make a note. This is your score.

2 – Push-ups

These can be performed from the knees OR from the toes - pick the progression level that is appropriate for you, and stay consistent during testing throughout the program.

Elbows and upper arm break parallel . . . body stays in a totally straight line, no hip sag or "A-frame" . . . no adjusting the knees, hands, or feet during the test. Body cannot touch the floor at the bottom of a rep; cannot lock out and rest at the top.

Do a single, unbroken set of as many as you can. This is your score.

3 – Pull-ups

Option one: the Flexed Arm Hang. Pull yourself or get help up, clearing the bar with the chin and cleanly touching the neck or chest at the top. Your palms should be facing towards you.

Hold this position as long as you can. Time yourself. The number of seconds you can hang with your chin over the bar unassisted is your score.

Option two: Standard Pull-ups. Pull-ups are done with an overhand grip. Start fully hanging from the bar, with arms fully extended. Pull yourself up, clearing the bar with the chin and cleanly touching the neck or chest at the top. Slowly lower yourself down, under control, until arms are fully extended at the bottom.
Do a single, unbroken set of as many as you can. This is your score.

4 – Burpees

Thighs and torso much touch the ground at the bottom of the movement. Full extension of the body—knees, hips, and upper body—as well as a jump and clap of the hands over the head must be completed at the top of each rep.

Do as many reps as you can with perfect form in one minute. This is your score.

5 – One-Arm Kettlebell Press

The kettlebell is cheat curled or cleaned to the shoulder to get into starting position. Assume a rack position with the kettlebell so you can touch the thumb to the collar bone, and so the kettlebell is in contact with two additional points—the forearm and upper arm. The candidate's feet are in approximately a hip-width stance. The elbow will stay underneath the kettlebell at the weight is pressed overhead. The torso and legs stay static during the entire movement. The heels stay down during the entire movement. The movement is complete at full arm extension. The kettlebell is returned to the ground in the same fashion it was picked up.

Press as heavy a 'bell as you can on either side for a single rep. This is your score.

PROGRAM OVERVIEW

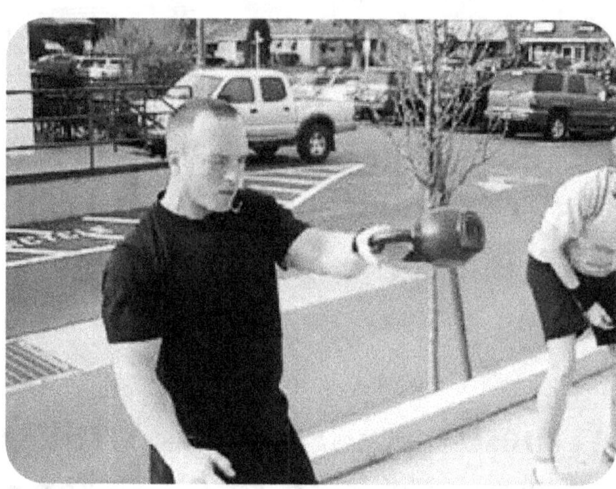

The CORE Kettlebell Challenge is a performance-based program.

See, training for a body composition goal—such as "losing ten pounds in six weeks" or something similar—is perfectly fine.

But what I've seen in training thousands and thousands of clients over the years is that it's not particularly motivating.

I also feel this way on a personal level. I know that if I just work out to "stay fit", and have no particular specific goal I'm working towards, I will get lazy and fat and out of shape.

But if I have a performance-based goal—as we do with this program, with the testing and the workouts themselves—it keeps me motivated, plus I lose fat and gain strength and get into and stay in great physical shape, all at the same time. And the same seems to hold true for my clients.

Now. I believe forty days is the perfect amount of time to get fantastic results yet stay focused, because there is an end to the program in sight. The workouts are simple and straightforward, yet quite challenging. They are also backed by science. According to the President's Council on Sports, Fitness and Nutrition, adults should do at least 75 minutes per week of "strenuous" cardiovascular activity (what we're doing with the CORE Kettlebell Challenge workouts), and at least two times per week of strength training.

We satisfy both of these requirements with workouts that last around twenty minutes, performed three to four times per week.

And the setup is SUPER simple. **You're just going to make your way through the training plan, starting with workout one, and do a workout every other day for six weeks. You'll end up doing twenty kettlebell workouts total.**

You are also going to run or walk a 5K two additional days per week, for a total of five to six days per week of exercise. This is also based on the President's Council on Sports, Fitness and Nutrition recommendation for "moderate" cardiovascular activity. This is a very simple way to work on your aerobic base and get some additional activity that will not dip into recovery and impact your kettlebell workouts. See the FAQ section in the back of the book for additional information and tips on this portion of the workout.

<u>So your week one will look like this:</u>

Monday – Kettlebell Workout 1
Tuesday – Run/Walk 5K
Wednesday – Kettlebell Workout 2
Thursday – Run/Walk 5K
Friday – Kettlebell Workout 3
Saturday – Off
Sunday – Kettlebell Workout 4

On Warming Up

Pick one of the warm up sequences to do before each kettlebell workout. Go at an easy pace and get your body physically and mentally prepared for the work to come. We'll hit some common "problem" areas (knees, hips, core, shoulders), and practice some of the movement patterns you will encounter in your main workout for the day.

On Recommended Weights

For all of the kettlebell exercises, I have put "recommended weights". This is a starting point to give you a ballpark idea of where you should start. If you are just getting into things and want to start light, feel free to bump the weights down. If you are more advanced and really want to go for it, use heavier weights. Also see the section on recommended weights in the Q&A part of the book for more details.

Warm Up #1: Do as many reps as you can of each exercise in **30 seconds**; no rest between moves; do **two rounds total**:

Run in Place
Bodyweight Squats
Plank Hold
Recline Rows

Warm Up #2: Do as many reps as you can of each exercise in **30 seconds**; no rest between moves; do **two rounds total**:

Jumping Jacks
Bodyweight Squats
Push Ups
Recline Rows

Warm Up #3: Do as many reps as you can of each exercise in **30 seconds**; no rest between moves; do **two rounds total**:

Run in Place
Lunges
Plank Hold
One-Arm Kettlebell Rows (recommended weight = 8k women / 16k men)

Kettlebell Challenge Workout #1: "The Machine" – Complete as many rounds as possible of the circuit below in **20** minutes:

50 Jumping Jacks

10 One-Arm Kettlebell Swings (right side) (recommended weight = 8k women / 16k men)

10 Burpees

10 One-Arm Kettlebell Swings (left side) (recommended weight = 8k women / 16k men)

Kettlebell Challenge Workout #2: "Beast" – **4** rounds, **45** seconds on, **15**-second rest between moves, **1**-minute rest between rounds:

Kettlebell Swings (recommended weight = 16k women / 24k men)

Push-Ups

Lunges

Pull-Ups OR Recline Rows

Burpees

Kettlebell Challenge Workout #3: "Animal" – Complete **5** rounds of the circuit below for time:

7 Burpees

7 One-Arm Kettlebell Swings (per side) (recommended weight = 8k women / 16k men)

20 Kettlebell Squats (recommended weight = 8k women / 16k men)

10 Lunges

Kettlebell Challenge Workout #4: "Hollywood" – **5** rounds, **30** seconds on, **15**-second rest between moves, **1**-minute rest between rounds

One-arm Kettlebell Swings (15 seconds per side) (recommended weight = 8k women / 16k men)

One-Arm Kettlebell Presses (15 seconds per side) (recommended weight = 8k women / 16k men)

Lunges (30 seconds per side)

One-Arm Kettlebell Rows (15 seconds per side) (recommended weight = 8k women / 16k men)

Jumping Jacks

Kettlebell Challenge Workout #5: "Bloodsport" – Complete as many rounds as possible of the circuit below in **20** minutes:

10 Lunges (right side)
10 One-Arm Kettlebell Swings (per side) (recommended weight = 8k women / 16k men)
10 Lunges (left side)
30 Jumping Jacks

Kettlebell Challenge Workout #6: "Cyborg" – **4** rounds, **45** seconds on, **15**-second rest between moves, **1**-minute rest between rounds:

Kettlebell Squats (recommended weight = 8k women / 16k men)
Plank Hold
Lunges
Burpees
High knees

Kettlebell Challenge Workout #7: "Street Fighter" – 20 minutes AMRAP (As Many Rounds as Possible)

10 Burpees

5 One-Arm Kettlebell Presses (right side) (recommended weight = 8k women / 16k men)

10 Push-Ups

5 One-Arm Kettlebell Presses (left side) (recommended weight = 8k women / 16k men)

Kettlebell Challenge Workout #8: "Maximum Risk" – 5 rounds, 30 seconds on, 15-second rest between moves, 1-minute rest between rounds

Kettlebell Squats (recommended weight = 8k women / 16k men)

Plank Hold

Lunges

One-Arm Kettlebell Rows (15 seconds per side) (recommended weight = 8k women / 16k men)

High Knees

Kettlebell Challenge Workout #9: "The Terminator" – EMOTM (every minute on the minute) for **20** minutes

Minute 1 – Kettlebell Swings – 20 (recommended weight = 16k women / 24k men)
Minute 2 – Push-Ups – 15
Minute 3 – Burpees – 8

Kettlebell Challenge Workout #10: "Cold Steel" – **4** rounds, **45** seconds on, **15**-second rest between moves, **1**-minute rest between rounds

Kettlebell swings (recommended weight = 16k women / 24k men)
Push-Ups
Kettlebell Squats (recommended weight = 8k women / 16k men)
Pull-Ups OR Recline Rows
Jumping Jacks

Kettlebell Challenge Workout #11: "Mind of a Lunatic" – 5 rounds, 30 seconds on, 15-second rest between moves, 1-minute rest between rounds:

One-Arm Kettlebell Swings (22.5 seconds per side) (recommended weight = 8k women / 16k men)
Push-Ups
Kettlebell Squats (recommended weight = 8k women / 16k men)
One-Arm Kettlebell Presses (22.5 seconds per side) (recommended weight = 8k women/16k men)
Burpees

Kettlebell Challenge Workout #12: "Megatron" – 5 rounds, 30 seconds on, 15-second rest between moves, 1-minute rest between rounds:

Kettlebell Squats (recommended weight = 8k women / 16k men)
Plank Hold
Lunges
One-arm Kettlebell Rows (recommended weight = 8k women / 16k men)
High Knees in Place

Kettlebell Challenge Workout #13: "Pandemonium" – 20 minutes
AMRAP (As Many Rounds as Possible)

5 Burpees

12 Kettlebell Swings (recommended weight = 16k women / 24k men)

10 Lunges (per side)

10 One-Arm Kettlebell Rows (per side) (recommended weight = 8k women / 16k men)

10 Push-Ups

Kettlebell Challenge Workout #14: "Tank" – 4 rounds, 45 seconds on, 15-second rest between moves, 1-minute rest between rounds

One-Arm Kettlebell Swings (22.5 seconds per side) (recommended weight = 8k women / 16k men)

Plank Hold

Kettlebell Squats (recommended weight = 8k women / 16k men)

Pull-Ups OR Recline Rows

Burpees

Kettlebell Challenge Workout #15: "Bull Durham" – 20 minutes
AMRAP (As Many Rounds as Possible)

15 Kettlebell Swings (recommended weight = 16k women / 24k men)

10 Lunges (per side)

12 One-Arm Kettlebell Rows (per side) (recommended weight = 8k women / 16k men)

50 Jumping Jacks

Kettlebell Challenge Workout #16: "Fancy Pants" – 5 rounds, **30** seconds on, **15**-second rest, **1**-minute rest between rounds

Kettlebell Squats (recommended weight = 8k women / 16k men)

Plank Hold

Lunges (30 seconds per side)

One-Arm Kettlebell Rows (15 seconds per side) (recommended weight = 8k women / 16k men)

High Knees

Kettlebell Challenge Workout #17: "Metamorphosis" – 2 rounds for time:

30 Jumping Jacks

10 Burpees

30 High Knees

30 Recline Rows

30 Jumping Jacks

8 Lunges per side

30 High Knees

10 One-Arm Kettlebell Swings per side (recommended weight = 8k women / 16k men)

30 Jumping Jacks

30 Bodyweight Squats

Kettlebell Challenge Workout #18: "Battle Cry" – 5 rounds, 45 seconds on, 15-second rest, 1 minute between rounds

Lunges

Burpees

One-Arm Kettlebell Rows (22.5 seconds per side) (recommended weight = 8k women / 16k men)

One-Arm Kettlebell Presses (22.5 seconds per side) (recommended weight = 8k women/16k men)

Kettlebell Challenge Workout #19: "Gunslingers" – 20 minutes AMRAP (As Many Rounds as Possible)

5 One-Arm Kettlebell Presses (right side) (recommended weight = 8k women / 16k men)
5 One-Arm Kettlebell Presses (left side) (recommended weight = 8k women / 16k men)
10 Burpees
15 Recline Rows
10 Lunges (per leg - 20 total)

Kettlebell Challenge Workout #20: "Sixth Sense" – 5 rounds, **30** seconds on, **15**-second rest, **1**-minute rest between rounds

Kettlebell Swings (recommended weight = 16k women / 24k men)
Burpees
Pull-Ups OR Recline Rows
One-Arm Kettlebell Presses (recommended weight = 8k women / 16k men)

PART 3

Q&A

Come back with your shield—or on it.

—Plutarch, Moralia No. 241

COMMON KETTLEBELL QUESTIONS AND ANSWERS

Now you have everything you need for success.

You have the tested, proven, six-week kettlebell program for fat loss—at ANY age.

But maybe you have questions about specifics.

That's why I put together this FAQ section.

I've made my best attempt to answer the most frequent questions we get about kettlebell training in my daily interactions.

Hope this helps!

QUESTION: I know WHAT to do. I just have trouble DOING it on a regular basis. How do I stay motivated to work out?

Here is what can be an all-too-common pattern:

You get all fired up and set some goals.

You're going to work out every morning. Or cut out the after-dinner snacking! Or drop the two beers every night. Or whatever else . . .

. . . and you do great, for a little while . . . But then one, two, three weeks in, you fall into your old habits . . . and you feel like you're right back where you started.

Clearly, there are a LOT of factors at play here.

So I'm just going to tell you what works for ME.

See, six or seven years ago, I was super, super focused on work.

I was driving like a maniac, and that's pretty much what I thought about all day, every day.

How can I get better, how can I succeed, how can I grow my business?

At that time, my workouts and nutrition were all about optimizing my performance so I could get a little more productivity and that extra "edge."

So if this is *your* current season of life, maybe that's YOUR reason why.

OR maybe you're in a phase similar to the one that I am currently. I do think about work and improving the business and growing, don't get me wrong . . . but now my family is also my priority.

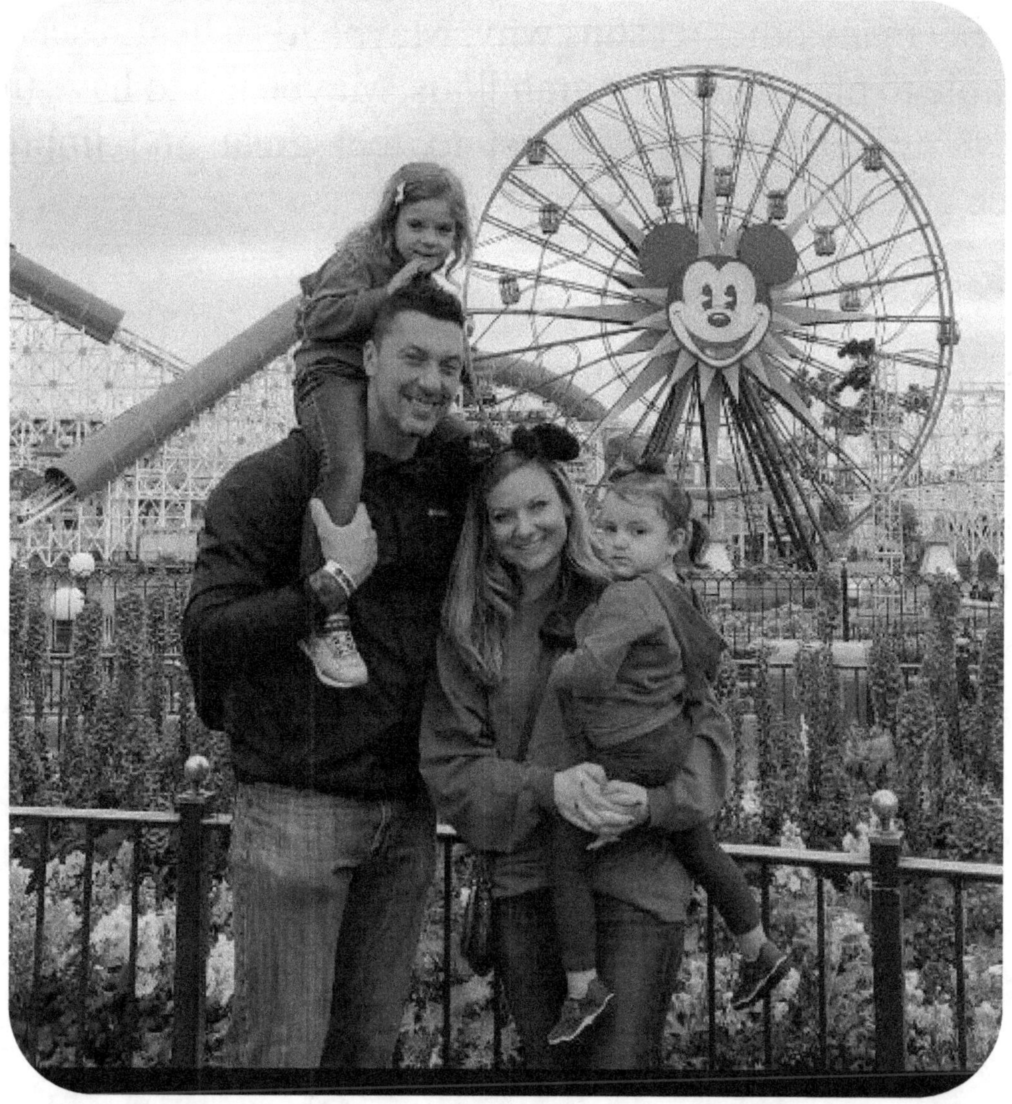

So now it's about balancing out providing for them with also being able to spend time with them.

Balancing out work with health because I want to be around for them, for a long time to come.

This is a HUGE motivation when maybe I don't feel like working out, or cutting back on the beers, or getting to bed early, or whatever else.

And if you are in a similar time of life, maybe this is your "reason why" too.

There are SO many other reasons why. Maybe it's a health scare. Maybe it's to be able to play with your grandkids. Maybe it's to have the energy and zeal to travel. Maybe it's just to feel great and improve your confidence and change your outlook on life.

And no reasons are right or wrong.

They are right for YOU—and that's all the matters.

Bottom line, I hope today's message gets you thinking, and possibly spurs you to action.

QUESTION: I need help with my diet! What should I eat while following this program?

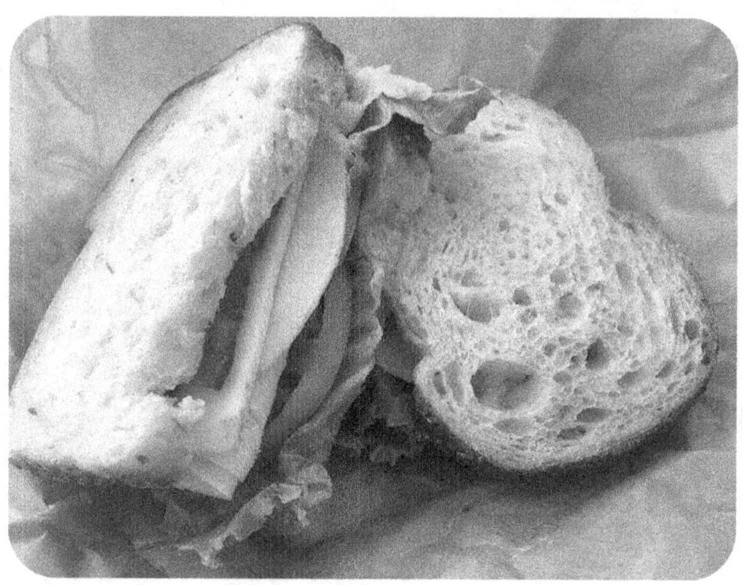

When it comes to following a diet plan, some people do better following a very specific plan.

Visit ForestVance.com and check out the "official" FVT diet plan there.

This book is specifically focused on kettlebell training, so I am trying to go an inch wide and a mile deep on just that topic.

However, here are the "Rules of Lean Eating" we preach daily at our training studios.

These rules are largely based on one of the most well-known research studies on long-term weight loss maintenance (Montesi, El Gosch, Brodosi et. al. 2016).

Follow these rules, and you've got the core of healthy nutrition.

FVT Rules of Lean Eating

Eat Lean Protein at Every Meal

Include a lean protein source at every meal. This could be poultry, fish, egg(s), protein powder, etc.

Eat Veggies and/or Fruits at Every Meal

Your primary carbohydrate source should be veggies and/or fruits. Your goal is to include one of these at every meal.

Eat a "Good" Fat at Every Meal

Finish off each meal with a "dash" of good fat, like nuts, seeds, olive oil, avocado, etc.

Minimize Your Starches and Processed Carbohydrates

Keep your intake of things like bread, pasta, crackers, etc. to a minimum.

REALLY Minimize Your Sugar Intake

Rarely, if ever, eat sugar. Period.

Drink About Half of Your Body Weight in Ounces of Water Per Day

So if you weigh 150 pounds, you should shoot for drinking about 75 ounces of water per day (nine or ten 8-ounce glasses).

Follow the 90 Percent Rule

This rule says that you need to be "on" with the seven rules 90 percent of the time to see progress.

For example, if you eat three times per day, seven days per week . . . no more than two of your meals can break these rules.

You CAN go off the plan everyone once in a while . . . it's just what you do on a regular and consistent basis that will determine your ultimate results.

Simple, right?

But if you just follow these seven rules 90 percent of the time, you're almost guaranteed to get to your ideal weight in a short amount of time.

QUESTION: I can't run. What can I do instead of running a 5K?

You can walk. You can jog. You can run. Do the intensity that is right for YOU.

The important thing here is that we are trying to get what we'd call "moderate-intensity" cardiovascular activity. It's not high intensity - we are saving that for the kettlebell workouts. These are extra movement sessions to train your heart, burn fat, and live a generally active lifestyle.

Another thing you can try, that I have personally had GREAT success with, is the run-walk-run method. This method was developed by Jeff Galloway. You can check out his book in the Works Referenced section at the back of this book. But the idea is that you run and then walk at a specific interval, from the very beginning of your run.

For me, it's made a huge difference. I can run much longer without pain, and my recovery time is much faster. Check out his book for the full details, but the timing looks something like this:

- Walkers: shuffle for 30 seconds after 2 to 4 minutes of walking
- 14-minute mile pace: alternate 1 minute running/1 minute walking
- 12-minute mile pace: alternate 2 minutes running/1 minute walking
- 10-minute mile pace: alternate 3 minutes running/1 minute walking
- 8-minute mile pace: alternate 4 minutes running/30 seconds walking

QUESTION: Can I do extra workouts/combine this with another routine?

Yes, BUT, you need to be strategic in how you do it.

Do NOT just double up on some other workouts, with no rhyme or reason.

Because recovery is very important, and it could make or break your success with this program.

Here's where I would start:

1. Add in some "off-day" flexibility/mobility/recovery work. You could do something like a full sixty- to ninety-minute yoga class on an "off" day (that's what I frequently do), and/or you could add five to ten minutes of mobility work in the mornings to start your day. (Check out ForestVance.com for a full program for this.)

2. You could add in extra conditioning work. You could sub out your 5K run/walks with something else longer or more intense. And/or you could add an extra/different conditioning workout. (I have a program dedicated to this at ForestVance.com. Go there to check it out.)

3. You could add extra lifting using my Barbell Basics program. It's designed to be "bolted on" to a program like this. The lifts are done after your warm-up, before your main kettlebell/bodyweight workout for the day. Check out ForestVance.com for that program too.

<u>QUESTION: What is the best time of day to work out?</u>

The best time is the time that you are most likely to do it.

For elite athletes, the answer to this question might be different. Your body might be optimized to perform the best at a specific time. Or maybe you are preparing for an event that is actually taking place at a specific time of day and you want to prepare yourself mentally and physically for that.

For most people, showing up and doing the workouts on a regular basis day in, day out, for a long period of time, is the main challenge.

The biggest key is to look at the rest of your life and figure out times during the week where you can be the most consistent.

<u>QUESTION: What brand of kettlebells do you recommend?</u>

There are a lot of great kettlebell brands out there these days.

For the last gym we outfitted, we purchased kettlebells from Rep Fitness.

I got these on Amazon.com. They are nice quality and very reasonably priced.

Also, there is a big difference between competition 'bells and cast-iron ones.

For Hardstyle kettlebell training, like we do in the CORE Kettlebell Challenge, cast iron are great.

If you were going to compete in Girevoy sport, the sport of competitive kettlebell lifting, the competition kettlebells are best because they are all the same size and they are designed for the specific demands of that sport.

QUESTION: What are the best shoes to wear for kettlebell workouts?

When training with kettlebells, the best option is to go with no shoes.

This will allow you to connect to the ground properly and have a great foot position while training.

It allows you to most efficiently transfer energy generated from the ground to the upper body.

And more.

However, there are times—if you are training outside, for example, and don't want to cut your feet—that you will need to wear shoes.

In this case, something with a flat sole is your best bet.

So you want stiff, flat-soled shoes, so you can get as close to barefoot as possible.

QUESTION: Is it okay to wear gloves during kettlebell workouts?

I do not recommend wearing gloves while training with kettlebells. Here are four great reasons why:

1. The gloves can keep the kettlebell from moving around the hand properly. Especially if you are doing higher-rep ballistic moves where the 'bell rotates around your hand multiple times—cleans, snatches, etc.—the gloves will really get in the way.

2. If you DO try to attempt to use gloves and get into serious kettlebell training as described in reason 1, the gloves can actually "bunch up" and end up digging into your hands even MORE.

3. Gloves can hinder the sensory connection from the hands to the brain. You won't feel what the weight is doing and exactly what is happening during your workout, and it won't be as good.

4. They look kind of lame—so tough it out.

QUESTION: What is the reason for chalking one's hands when using kettlebells?

The purpose for chalking one's hands when using kettlebell is to improve your grip.

If your hands become slippery, you lose your grip—and chalk helps with this.

Think of it like sweat control.

It also can keep the hands cool and can keep the hands from tearing.

It's also a personal preference: some people use it, some don't, both end up doing fine.

One important thing: you only need a little bit. Just enough to coat your hands is perfect. More is not better, and it also makes a huge mess.

QUESTION: What size kettlebells should I start with?

I remember my first kettlebell workout like it was yesterday.

It was 2006 . . . my training partner at the time brought in his 35-pound kettlebell to use with our workout for the day . . . and I chuckled.

I was—and am—fairly strong . . . I was probably benching around 350 at the time, squatting 425 or 450, and deadlifting around 500 . . . and I thought, what is a little 35-pound weight going to do for me?

BOY was I wrong! We got a couple of minutes into the little finisher he had planned for us with the kettlebell, and I was smoked.

I couldn't believe the total body workout you could get with this little kettlebell, in such a short amount of time.

And so, as what weight to start with, I would say:

- A 16k (35 pound) and 24k (53 pound) for men
- An 8k (18 pound) and 16k (35 pound) for women

If you're a total beginner and / or want to ease into things, you could start lighter than this.

If you're more advanced and confident in starting with heavier weights, you could bump up.

But this guideline is a great starting point for most men and women getting started with kettlebells.

Wrap-Up and What's Next

Men and women need to know that they CAN get stronger, lose the fat, and feel great - at ANY age.

This program is the culmination of 23 years of in-the-trenches training and hands-on experience. From my early days of learning to lift weights for high school football and track, to evolving and growing to over three hundred pounds for college football and a "cup of coffee" in the NFL, to the last fifteen years of my strength journey working in the fitness industry—it's all here.

Using kettlebell "blast" workouts that take about twenty minutes, three to four times per week, you are going to get AMAZING results.

And I can't wait to hear about them!

If you love this program, I also suggest you check out my other books, training courses, and coaching programs at my website, ForestVance.com. I have programs you can do after you're done with this one, programs that complement this one, and much more.

Here's to your success -

Forest Vance
Master of Science, Human Movement
Certified Kettlebell Instructor
ForestVance.com

Works Referenced

Baechle, Thomas R. *Essentials of Strength Training and Conditioning*. Human Kinetics, 2016.

Burns, Brian, et al. *Yoga for Beginners*. Rosen Pub., 2012.

Ferriss, Timothy. *The 4-Hour Body: an Uncommon Guide to Rapid Fat-Loss, Incredible Sex, and Becoming Superhuman*. Harmony Books, 2012.

Foster C, Farland CV, Guidotti F, et al. The Effects of High Intensity Interval Training vs Steady State Training on Aerobic and Anaerobic Capacity. *J Sports Sci Med*. 2015;14(4):747–755. Published 2015 Nov 24.

Galloway, Jeff. *The Run Walk Method*. Meyer & Meyer Sport, 2016.

HHS Office, and Council on Sports. "Physical Activity Guidelines for Americans." HHS.gov, US Department of Health and Human Services, 1 Feb. 2019, **www.hhs.gov/fitness/be-active/physical-activity-guidelines-for-americans/index.html**.

Montesi L, El Ghoch M, Brodosi L, Calugi S, Marchesini G, Dalle Grave R. Long-term weight loss maintenance for obesity: a multidisciplinary approach. *Diabetes Metab Syndr Obes*. 2016;9:37–46. Published 2016 Feb 26. doi:10.2147/DMSO.S89836

Schoenfeld, Brad & Contreras, Bret. (2014). The Muscle Pump: Potential Mechanisms and Applications for Enhancing Hypertrophic Adaptations. Strength and Conditioning Journal. 36. 21-25. 10.1097/SSC.0000000000000021.

Sears, Barry. *The Zone Diet: 150 Fast and Simple Healthy Recipes from the Bestselling Author of The Zone" and "Mastering the Zone".* Thorsons, 1999.

Somerset, Dean. "The World's Easiest Assessment and How to Instantly Tell If You Need More Mobility." *DeanSomerset.com*, 3 May 2016, deansomerset.com/the-worlds-easiest-assessment-and-how-to-tell-if-you-need-more-mobility-instantly

TSATSOULINE, PAVEL. *ENTER THE KETTLEBELL!: Strength Secret of the Soviet Supermen.* Dragon Door Publications Inc., 2018.

Verstegen, Mark, et al. *Core Performance: the Revolutionary Workout Program to Transform Your Body and Your Life.* Rodale, 2007.

Wade, Paul. *Convict Conditioning: How to Bust Free of All Weakness Using the Lost Secrets of Supreme Survival Strength.* Dragon Door Publications Inc., 2018.

How to Get Dozens of Advanced, Fat-Burning, Muscle-Building, Kettlebell Workouts—Each for Less Than the Cost of a Personal Training Session

Now you can get almost an endless supply of fat-blasting, muscle-building kettlebell workouts. I've put all of my best-selling training plans together in one place. Visit my website at ForestVance.com to check them out.

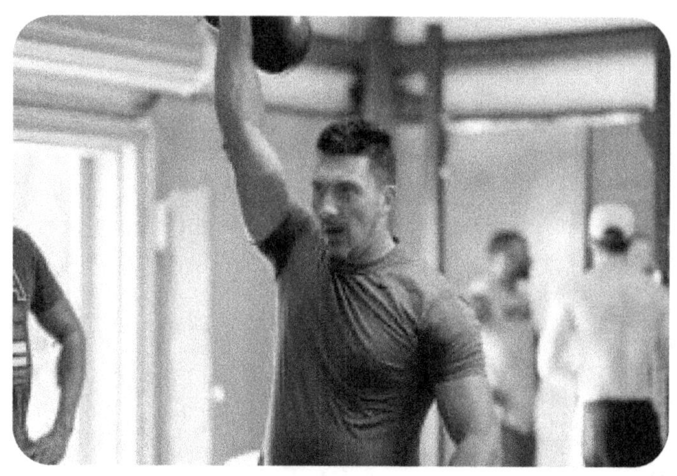

You'll find more advanced kettlebell programs like this one, for both fat loss and muscle gain . . . "hybrid" training workouts where you'll learn how to blend more traditional barbell work with kettlebells so you can get big AND strong AND athletic, all at the same time . . . bodyweight workouts to help you both lose fat and gain muscle, using little or even zero equipment . . . programs for extreme cardio conditioning and recovery, and more.

No matter your current goal or problem with reaching it, I have a program for you.

Visit my website at ForestVance.com to see my full product library today.